WHAT ADOLESCENTS OUGHT TO KNOW

WHAT ADOLESCENTS OUGHT TO KNOW

Sexual Health Texts in Early Twentieth-Century America

JENNIFER BUREK PIERCE

UNIVERSITY OF MASSACHUSETTS PRESS

Amherst and Boston

LC 2011012390
ISBN 978-1-55849-892-1 (paper)
ISBN 978-1-55849-891-4 (library cloth)

Designed by Sally Nichols
Set in Ivory and ITC Galliard
Printed and bound by Thomson-Shore, Inc.

Library of Congress Cataloging-in-Publication Data

Burek Pierce, Jennifer.
  What adolescents ought to know : sexual health texts in early twen-
tieth-century America / Jennifer Burek Pierce.
    p. cm. — (Print culture and the history of the book)
  ISBN 978-1-55849-892-1 (paper : alk. paper) — ISBN 978-1-55849-891-4
(library cloth : alk. paper) 1. Sex instruction for teenagers—United
States—History—20th century—Sources. 2. Sex instruction for
teenagers—France—History—20th century—Sources. 3. Fournier,
Alfred, 1832–1914. 4. Sexual health—Study and teaching—United
States—History—20th century—Sources. 5. Sexually transmitted diseases—United States—Prevention—History—20th century—Sources.
6. Teenagers—Sexual behavior—United States—History—20th century—Sources. 7. Teenagers—Health and hygiene—United States—
History—20th century—Sources. 8. Teenagers—Books and reading—United States—History—20th century—Sources. 9. Written
communication—United States—History—20th century. 10. Books
and reading—United States—History—20th century. I. Title.
  HQ57.2.B87 2011
  306.70835—dc22

                                                    2011012390

British Library Cataloguing in Publication data are available.

For J. Louise Malcomb, Bethany Templeton Klem,
and librarians everywhere

CONTENTS

ILLUSTRATIONS

ACKNOWLEDGMENTS

This manuscript has had a long genesis. From my first encounters with the seemingly strident convictions of librarians whose concerns with children and vice filled the pages of old issues of *Library Journal* and *Public Libraries*, to the days I spent reading in the Kinsey Institute library in an effort to make sense of nineteenth-century physicians' horror of books and disease alike, it has been a literal and metaphorical journey. I have logged hours sitting in libraries, and in cars and airplanes, too, to reach the far-away places holding papers necessary to ravel the threads of the story that I first glimpsed in libraries in Bloomington, Indiana. Hours have been spent, not only in research and writing, but in conversation with people who have supported the development of this project, whether in formal or informal colloquies.

A number of institutions and organizations have invited me to share my research, providing opportunities to venture my sense of the connections and themes I saw emerging at various stages of this work. Among the first was the Medical Humanities Program at Indiana University–Purdue University Indianapolis, where Bill Schneider encouraged my participation in the centennial-driven historical analysis of the state's eugenics activities. At the University of Iowa, Susan C. Lawrence welcomed me and invited me to share my research on French hygiene pamphlets with the school's Society for the History of Medicine. The faculty, staff, and students who comprise the University of Iowa's Center for the Book have also, through their Book Studies Seminar and many other interactions, sustained my efforts to understand the processes of dissemination and the significance of these texts. Also at Iowa, my colleague André Brock and others asked insightful questions about my research during a Project on the Rhetoric of Inquiry colloquium, after I had moved from the initial identification of texts to the issues that would inform this manuscript. The Department of Telecommunications at Indiana University also asked me to share this work in its later stages.

My debt to librarians is considerable, not least because I was born to and raised by one. My graduate assistants, who have gone on to libraries of their own, have provided research support, from tracking down errant source material to proofreading; Melissa Groveman and Anne Marie Moser supported the initial research, and Elizabeth Boyne has seen the project through its later stages. Steve Tatum, while a graduate student at the University of Iowa, doggedly pursued some of the articles that would ultimately allow me to see my subjects in human terms. At libraries, archives, and research centers across the nation, library and information professionals have generously given their time and their knowledge to enrich my work. At the Kinsey Institute in Bloomington, Indiana, Shawn Wilson has unfailingly made space for me and located materials for this project. The Lilly Library, also at Indiana University, and the Indiana State archives accommodated my research with courtesy. At the University of Iowa, Ed Holtum has shared the resources of the John Martin Rare Books Room in the Hardin Library for Health Sciences, while David Schoonover and Sid Huttner have facilitated my access to Special Collections materials. Among the other institutions that have provided pivotal resources, the Elmer L. Andersen Library at the University of Minnesota has been essential, and archivist David Klaassen and his staff aided my work considerably through their skillful organization of resources, knowledge of their holdings, and good cheer. Chris Lyons of the McGill University Osler History of Medicine Library, and Arlene Shaner and Miriam Mandelbaum of the New York Academy of Medicine's Library, have been more than kind. Matthew Sheehy of the New York Public Library, Ed Desrochers of the Phillips Exeter Academy Archives, Daniel Hope at Bowdoin College, and the Special Collections staff at Morris Library at Southern Illinois University, Carbondale, have answered questions and directed me to texts needed to connect the work of the various authors and reformers whom I have studied. I appreciate the aid of all who have spurred my research and constrained my inaccuracies.

Visiting far-away libraries requires financial support, and I am grateful to the Graduate College, International Programs, and the Old Gold Fellowship Program at the University of Iowa for funding which has allowed me to undertake the travel for this project. Further, the University's Office of the Vice President for Research has generously provided subvention funds in support of this publication.

I gratefully acknowledge permission to use, as the basis for Chapter 3, a biographical essay on John Hurty published in the *Indiana Magazine of History*.

Beyond the at times exotic and exhausting travels to give talks and to make use of unique resources, there is the continual, day-to-day effort to write sensibly about a complex array of texts, to draw out the story that these resources help to tell. Finding words to convey the critical facts, the reasonable conclusions, and the curiously engaging aspects of these sources has taken not only my time and effort, but that of friends and colleagues who have been willing to read drafts of this project as it has unfolded. Foremost among them has been Herb Snyder, whose willingness to wade through the verbal swamps of my words has considerably eased the burdens of readers who followed. I also am indebted to Jon Wilcox and Michael Bonin, who have listened to my explanations of this research, read drafts of chapters, and saw the sense in things, even when I doubted. Their confidence and encouragement has meant much to me. To David Nordloh, too, I am similarly grateful, not least because he recently directed me to Monty Python's "Novel Writing" skit on Thomas Hardy's composition of *The Return of the Native*. My editor, Brian Halley, and others affiliated with University of Massachusetts Press have patiently and carefully seen this work through its final stages.

Finally, it falls to recognize two individuals without whose essential contributions this project would have been much different, and much more difficult, if indeed it could have been done at all. Bethany Templeton Klem worked as my graduate assistant while the book-length version of this research took shape, and her gracious assistance of every sort eased my way. Lou Malcomb, during my time in her Government Documents class and afterward, gently persisted in explaining the need for research on the untold stories behind Indiana government publications. Her library was where this all began.

WHAT ADOLESCENTS
OUGHT TO KNOW

INTRODUCTION

In 1901, Dr. Alfred Fournier committed an act both profoundly simple and strikingly revolutionary: he wrote a treatise on sexual and reproductive health for young men, full of cautions and information based on his clinical work at a leading Paris hospital. The publication, *Pour nos fils,* reflected Fournier's understanding of the threat represented by syphilis and gonorrhea and urged his adolescent readers to protect themselves against these diseases. The weapon he offered them was abstinence; the reward he promised was a future with a happy, healthy family. If this fifty-page booklet aided adolescent understanding of health and the body, it also encouraged Fournier's fellow reformers around the world to follow his lead in sharing current medical knowledge with the public.

It was not long before *Pour nos fils* became available to readers in at least a dozen countries, and within a decade, numerous prevention-oriented health tracts for young people were published. The rapid development of this genre is evident in market analysts' recognition of it as a measurable portion of the American book market by 1913. This growing body of literature would be translated and reprinted for distribution abroad, so that the same work could be purchased for young people in Providence, Rhode Island and in Punjab, India. Although linked by recent medical knowledge that sexually transmitted infection constituted a grave threat, the resulting publications were seldom strictly homogeneous, as some emphasized moralistic warnings while others opened windows into contemporary research on disease prevention. These transnational exchanges produced competing understandings of adolescence and sexuality in the early twentieth century, even as they aligned for the common purpose of preventing the spread of then-incurable disease.

There have been histories of sexually transmitted infection, histories of sexuality, and histories of adolescence in the United States.[1] These narratives of the ways that people once regarded sex and the health and moral issues it entailed have tended to emphasize a nationalist story. This treatment obscures the fuller narrative of early twentieth-century health research and reform, particularly its dependence on print culture, which made the exchange of information across borders possible. Extant scholarship on the campaign against syphilis on American shores de-emphasizes the transnational concerns and connections that developed along with the professed aim of preventing sexually transmitted infection in the Progressive Era. These prior studies consider morality the complement of contemporary medicine's shortcomings and seldom examine the implications of the uses of literacy in disease prevention efforts, much less the treatment-oriented research that continued well beyond the 1909 discharge of Dr. Paul Erlich's magic bullet, Salvarsan.

Scholarly scrutiny of the attention given to soldiers and sailors has prevailed, although many reformers sought to reach the ordinary adolescent, whom they understood as newly experiencing both sexual desire and freedom from the protections of home or school. As news coverage of the 1899 International Conference for the Prevention of Syphilis and Venereal Disease observed, "One of the points most insisted on, and the subject of a special recommendation, was that the youth of all countries should be instructed in the true significance of venereal disease, and the consequences that immediately and remotely pursue its victims."[2] Health campaigns orchestrated by the military sought the attention of male readers, and texts produced for enlistees cast women either as immoral seductresses or as wholesome wives who would be harmed by a husband's association with faithless women presumed to carry sexually transmitted infections like syphilis. Some information producers, for all their inclination toward popular notions of femininity as either pure or debased, counted young women among readers who needed to understand the risks that physicians had recently identified.

Examining works intended for male and female readers involves attention to multiple publication venues. The implications of different sites of information delivery, which included private, government, and commercial entities, also have been little explored. Attention to these varied omissions is a principal object of this study. This focus involves the final years of the nineteenth century, continuing through the 1930s, in order to encompass Fournier's groundwork for his campaign and the final copyright date of Sylvanus Stall's internationally circulated books which formed part of a loose, yet complex, network that produced sexual health texts for adolescents.

Authors like Fournier and Stall were acknowledged leaders and, as professional men, were for the most part unimpeded in their own quests for information. The texts they and other contemporaries produced connected the domain of professional medical knowledge and that of ordinary adolescent readers, creating what scholars have tended to see as a decidedly imperfect information flow. My research endeavors not so much to look at issues of authority and power curtailing sexual knowledge as it seeks to understand the connections that fostered development of a transnational print culture dedicated to disseminating sexual health information for adolescent readers. As Daniel T. Rodgers has written of the Progressive Era, "The reconstruction of American social politics was of a part with movements of politics and ideas throughout the North Atlantic world that trade and capitalism had tied together."[3] Uncovering these linkages begins to bridge presumed divides in the health community of that time and shows how texts were used to reshape cultural notions of adolescent health. The revised perspective on science, sex, and adolescence in the early twentieth century gives attention to how these phenomena were reinterpreted in the interest of disease prevention and social reform. Ultimately, these contentious and emergent ideas were directed toward reconceptualizing health and reading.

Some scholars have tended to read this early twentieth-century response to sexually transmitted infection as a correlate to the late twentieth century's confrontation of the AIDS virus. Constructing this parallel, though, overlooks the eugenic concerns with population decline that motivated many early reformers; the role of religion in earlier guidance on sexual health has likewise been extracted from such comparisons. Finally, seeing the modern as a mirror of the past overlooks the gendered nature of these earlier communications. More than serving as a caveat against moral responses to medical dilemmas, Progressive Era sexual and reproductive health campaigns demonstrated the cultural tensions that arose from efforts to make developing technical information generated by the professional scientific community available to the common reader, particularly a reader who was him- or herself still in the process of maturing.

This ambitious endeavor required writers to envision the young reader in new ways, giving attention to the emerging concept of adolescence as a time of life characterized by change, including newfound sexuality. Progressive Era sexual and reproductive health tracts for young readers thus reflected the efforts of physicians and reformers to grapple with a second stream of developing research that recognized adolescence as a significant, distinctive, and vulnerable condition. The most influential thinker in this area, psychologist G. Stanley Hall, saw adolescence as a troubled and troubling time. This diagnosis, though, bolstered the aims of hygiene reformers. Hall insisted that adolescence, a turbulent interim between childhood and adulthood, was crucial to the future capacity for reproduction and family life. Preparing for these responsibilities, Hall argued, required intervention; it was guidance of this nature that Fournier and others intended to provide.

How could a young person, whose understanding of self and society was still forming, become convinced of the importance of rethinking received values about intimacy? What would convince a young person to avoid acting on impulse, on desire, even as such actions had become both possible and pressing? What norms should be employed in these arguments, when social and legal precedents warned against committing ideas about sex to print? How, in other words, could information about sex be made both decent and compelling? These were the challenges early twentieth-century health reformers confronted, when the ability to diagnose diseases like syphilis had outpaced doctors' ability to respond effectively to infection. In this context, information represented the best and truest prophylactic. Hundreds, if not thousands, of tracts and treatises were developed with the aim of preventing the spread of sexually transmitted infection; of those publications, several stand out as success stories from the perspective of information dissemination.

Some pamphlets and books that advised adolescents of the need to protect their reproductive health, though developed for a particular audience, reached readers well beyond their authors' original intentions. A handful of health treatises were translated, republished, and circulated to new readerships around the globe. Because the connections that fostered the exchange of these titles represented a new and significant convergence of print and scientific networks, tracing the linkages that resulted from these interactions has focused my research.[4] Among the works whose inception or eventual success, as measured by international redistribution, owed some degree of debt to Fournier were brochures produced by private reform societies, a pamphlet produced through a public/private partnership, a play that was subsequently rewritten as a novel, and commercially sold nonfiction books. Texts' influence reflected a belief that reproductive health information could protect young people and preserve national interests, like citizens' health and economic power. Despite such common ground and good intentions, the proliferation of health resources met with difficulties. The development from a single tract, written by a medical researcher and given away to anyone who might be convinced to read it, to a thriving commercial publishing industry, presents a history of the means by which sex education moved from private conversation to purchased text in the early twentieth century. The related story, of reading guidance, illuminates the connections between health and reading that became intrinsic to an emergent discourse on adolescence during the Progressive Era.

That there were, however, limits to what might be printed was revealed both by the endurance of the 1873 Comstock Act, which targeted a broad spectrum of potentially obscene matter, and by Fournier's own publications. The doctor was committed to understanding the treatments available to his patients, and the advent of arsenic-based therapeutics that promised to cure syphilis led him to write general audience treatises explaining the new medical facts. The society that distributed *Pour nos fils* and its companion title, *Pour nos filles,* neither printed Fournier's later works nor revised its adolescent-oriented literature. Many other publishers of what became known as hygiene literature likewise continued publicizing the existence of infection without indicating that a remedy was possible. Medicine moved forward, but much popular prevention literature held back as debate and research continued. The adolescent reader, in the first decades of the twentieth century, was not invited to assess the ways science responded to the diseases regarded as the demise of a young person's future. In the 1930s, however, this subtle conflict was, if not resolved, then engaged more directly. While *What Every Young Man Ought to Know*, even in its last printing in 1936, still did not mention Salvarsan, the following year, U.S. Secretary of Public Health Thomas Parran declared, in the pages of *Reader's Digest* magazine, that the public must understand syphilis. The novelty of sexual health information began to recede, and with it the transnational forces that had competed for teenaged readers for four decades.

Research Methods and Theoretical Considerations

In 1909, Indiana Public Health Secretary John Hurty demanded of his colleagues around the state, "Why not strive to prevent fire?" This query, the title of an article in the state's monthly health bulletin that insisted on the need for open communication about the devastating consequences of sexually transmitted infection, began my own inquiries nearly a century later.

I started my research with the understanding that all aspects of reproductive health, particularly sexually transmitted infection, were shrouded by concerns about modesty and propriety during the Progressive Era. This reticence was evinced by prominent health activists, among them the women who studied and provided maternal and infant health care in conjunction with the Sheppard-Towner Act of 1921. Advocates for Sheppard-Towner legislation, who had already raised ire because of their scrutiny of pregnancy and childbirth, avoided further mention of inflammatory subjects in their public communications, while acknowledging venereal disease as a threat to mothers and infants during professional meetings that were closed to the general public.[5] Why, then, did a public health official in Indiana decide the state's residents needed to know about syphilis? Why did a strident call for frankness about sexual health avoid using words like *sex, syphilis,* or even *infection* to name the issues in an article for fellow health professionals? And what resulted from this urgent, if euphemistic, call to action? Informed, perhaps naïvely, by the notion of an ur-text in literary studies, these questions about Hurty's publication prompted my journeys to numerous special libraries and archives.

Further scrutiny of Hurty's directives to Indiana public health officials revealed that under the auspices of his state agency, he published a prevention-oriented booklet called *Social Hygiene vs. the Sexual Plagues*. Certain that Hurty did not arrive at his conviction that sexual health was a critical public health matter in the relative isolation of early twentieth-century Indiana, I wanted to identify his discursive partners, the other individuals who shared his zeal. It turned out that these individuals, Progressive Era authors and publishers of hygiene literature, were more or less literally everywhere. Among the prolific men and women who committed sexual health advice to print, some were more influential than others, and the threads of a network among these individuals became evident. Hurty, then, could be identified as one figure in an emerging international movement to provide sexual and reproductive health information to adolescents.

Hurty alternately voiced triumph about the number of requests his office received for the treatise and bitter disappointment about lack of media interest in his cause. To understand the highs and lows of interest in *Social Hygiene vs. the Sexual Plagues* that he chronicled each month in the state's public health bulletin, I turned to the records his office maintained, now held by the Indiana State Archives. Hurty's outbound correspondence documented this period of his official life, and his letter books held significant hints about the demand for health information during this time. While it was impossible to validate his claims that his office once received more than one hundred requests for *Social Hygiene vs. the Sexual Plagues* on a single day, it was nonetheless evident that numerous individuals, within the state's borders and outside them, wanted his treatise. That petitioners from the territories of New Mexico and Arizona, from the eastern states of New York and Massachusetts, and from Germany and Australia all wrote asking for the title indicated that Hurty's imperative was very much a shared one.

Thus began an iterative process of examining historical health texts for adolescents, medical writings on sexually transmitted infection of the same period, and recent scholarship on the history of medicine and reform activity in the late Victorian and early Progressive eras, looking for further evidence of connections. In many respects, each chapter of this book required a somewhat different methodology, depending on an at times unpredictable array of primary sources. Sometimes, as in the case of Hurty's work, letters provided indications of the development and distribution of a publication—plus the obstacles confronted. For approximately two years Hurty worked on the release of *Social Hygiene vs. the Sexual Plagues,* a project that included lobbying and fundraising, hiring a traveling speaker, and generating publicity, and letters detailed that endeavor.

Hurty's accounts of his successes also directed my attention to mass-media coverage of sexual and reproductive health in the early twentieth century, as he would from time to time remark on favorable news reports following a talk he had given or complain to a correspondent that his efforts to interest an editor in *Social Hygiene vs. the Sexual Plagues* had come to nothing. Hurty's own writing, and many of the state and national articles, indicated that thorough study of published primary texts addressing the controversial issue of venereal disease had to account for what remained unarticulated. Just as Hurty used the metaphor of fire, other writers engaged the problems of teen sex and syphilis under the cover of indirect titles like "I Didn't Know" and "Unnecessary Blindness."[6] Whether it appeared in the *Indiana Bulletin of Public Health* or *Ladies' Home Journal,* an article whose title seemed vague or so general as to offer no real sense of its content frequently spoke to these sensitive issues. These contemporary writings confirmed scholars' pronouncements about the persistence of moralizing responses to sexually transmitted infection, yet suggested some individuals nonetheless furthered access to science-driven health information.

The records of the French Society for Sanitary and Moral Prophylaxis founded by Fournier also clarified issues in the creation of sexual health titles for adolescents. A secretary shared correspondence with the membership, so that news and requests from individuals were part of the context of the Society's deliberations. While Fournier's treatise, *Pour nos fils,* was discussed after its publication, the subsequent work for female readers, *Pour nos filles,* was printed in its entirety for members prior to a lengthy and heated consideration of its appropriateness for the intended audience (the inclusion of this short work in a full-length, hardbound volume likewise suggested yet another means by which the Society's titles reached those who would read and republish its tracts). Discussion of whether to publish a pamphlet for young women was cloaked under talks given the label "The Threat of Venereal Disease to the Working Class," which addressed the question, "Must we, yes or no, enlighten young people of the working class about venereal disease; and if yes, by what means and actions?"[7] As the Society debated its responsibilities and limitations, its concerns and aspirations, members introduced new medical findings, condemned the permissiveness of popular culture, and worried about legal issues and publication costs in sometimes ranging conversations. Thus, the official records of this private association elaborated the multiple contexts that influenced its texts, including subsequent efforts by an unaffiliated playwright to depict the consequences of ignorance on stage. Supplemented by analysis of bibliographic records for international libraries, the Society's proceedings also show the reach of the works it published, as well as the diffuse sources of information that affected the production of health treatises for male and female adolescents.

Not all publishers, however, left documents detailing the behind-the-scenes workings of their organizations. Instead, compilations of internal and external texts are necessary to reveal their successes, conflicts, and connections to others in the burgeoning social hygiene movement. Two for-profit publishers relying on the findings of medical researchers like Fournier were Sylvanus Stall, a Lutheran minister turned editor and publisher, and Winfield Scott Hall, a physician from Northwestern University who converted his official role in health promotion with the U.S. military into a secondary commercial enterprise. The records of presses that sold the books and pamphlets authored by these men did not survive. Discerning the impact of their works, then, depends on marketing pieces and reviews, as well as mentions in the work of others engaged in promoting adolescent sexual and reproductive health. James Secord has described this tracing of a text's reception through the trails left by advertisements, reviews, diary entries, and public cultural references as "literary replication."[8]

The ways that a text exists, not simply as an independent work but as acknowledged in other texts, contribute significantly to our understanding of the popularization of newly established medical ideas. When a cause or a cure for a dire health condition is discovered, its originator often receives a champion's accolades, as peers and the press share the promising news or the controversy that ensues. As physicians' attention turned from discovery to dissemination of information, leading authors and editors could still be discerned by others' compliments and complaints, by the reappearance of tropes and tested phrases. Such references make plain a rivalry between Stall and Hall, a mutual awareness that they competed for readers of hygiene texts, and suggest the ways these authors interacted with physicians, reformers, and others interested in the problems of adolescence and sexuality.

The texts that warned teens against the complications of venereal disease were, in effect, a popularization of recent medical research. Medical texts that explained the state of scientific understanding of venereal disease then form a necessary complement to any analysis of popular writing on sexual and reproductive health. It is simple and relatively straightforward to observe that works for young people were moralistic and sometimes less than frank. The question of whether information resources omitted accepted, scientifically determined facts is a more challenging one. Many of these titles originated years before Fritz Schaudinn and Erich Hoffman identified the *spirochaeta pallida* under a microscope, before the creation of the Wasserman test to identify this infectious microbe, and before Salvarsan's antidotal power was patented. Even after these landmark events, physicians remained concerned about the certainty of diagnosis and the efficacy of treatments for syphilis. Given scientific and medical limitations, authors' insistence on abstinence, or continence, as they called the practice of sexual restraint, was all but inevitable when sexual health treatises for adolescents emerged. Other social conditions also had implications for health messages devised for teens.

Proponents' ideals led them to adopt a point of view that seems, on the surface, in sync with a perspective on sexuality finally less taboo:

adolescents will fare better if informed about their bodies and repro-duction. In the abstract, the early enterprise of educating young people about sexuality and health may seem noble or forward-thinking, yet few authors and publishers would strike a twenty-first-century audi-ence as conventionally heroic. Instead, many present-day scholars have cast these influential individuals as somewhat blemished figures in nar-ratives of this health campaign, often because of attitudes that were acceptable then and regrettable now. My aim is to balance contempo-rary accounts of these writers' heroism, more recent academic vilifica-tions of their allegiance to the cultural norms of their time, and other information that grounded the arguments advanced in print. This examination acknowledges that many writers failed to reflect twenty-first-century ideals, even as they shared sexual and reproductive health information for young people. Doing so was innovative and shifted the conventions of both print culture and health communication.

Undeniably, the values that informed these efforts were complex and not always, in hindsight, admirable. Reform-oriented communica-tion about sexual health simultaneously advocated eugenics in the advice offered to young people. Religious tenets, particularly those that ascribed subordinate and self-sacrificing positions to women in the interest of family, pervaded these works. While disease was to be cur-tailed, births were not. Medical discussions from this time insisted that condoms, which many medical men seemed to regard with a degree of squeamishness, would protect against disease transmission but pre-vented pregnancy, too. They regarded contraception with a suspicion that exceeded their dread of prophylactics historically, though not con-temporarily, produced from animal intestines. Condoms were never mentioned in works for young people, and child-bearing was celebrated as a source of happiness and fulfillment; behind the closed doors of meeting rooms and in the pages of professional journals, reformers worried about the vigor of fighting forces and the health of workers who played a pivotal role in national economies. Self-promotion and financial gain also factored into the production of health treatises for adolescents as hygiene books entered the literary market place. While contextual sources demonstrate that physicians did not abandon the pursuit of more promising cures because abstinence prior to a monogamous marriage was advocated as the primary means of disease prevention, the existence of multiple motives complicates the assessment of these early twentieth-century sexual and reproductive health treatises for young people.

Scholarship on this significant period of medical and public health work has typically posited national, linguistic, and other barriers to the sharing of information and ideas. In introducing new primary texts to the study of the dissemination of health information to illuminate the centrality of adolescence and the connections among global groups of reformers, this project applies research methods associated with print culture and rhetoric to works in the history of medicine. The texts informing this study belong to a range of genres; they are books, pamphlets, letters, government documents, medical treatises, advertisements, news reports, and ephemera. The conventions of each mode of discourse both shed light on and shadow issues in the development of hygiene treatises.

Collectively, the works that advised adolescents about threats to their sexual and reproductive health and the documents that provide insights into the creation and distribution of this literature reveal transnational interests in shaping the adolescent reader's health and sexuality. Where such views coalesced, texts were recirculated, and when notions of morality or science were in conflict, new writings were put forth to be distributed in turn. All of these resources, now more than a century old, depend on rich and at times curious vocabularies. Roger Chartier has observed that "by their choices and comparisons, historians assign new meaning to speech pulled out of the silence of the archives."[9] This process of constructing meaning, Chartier argues, is subject to principles of intention, truth, and verification. Consequently, I have read one document against another, contrasted one historical actor's views with his peers' perspectives, with the aim of being able to represent long-ago events critically and accurately; this negotiation of meaning through the interplay of many and diverse sources is intended to bring us closer to understanding what prompted the intersection of social and professional interests in sex, science, and adolescence at a pivotal time.

It might seem tempting or even natural to impose Foucault's reading of historical discourse about sexuality onto the early twentieth-century medical mandate to share information about reproduction with adolescents. The texts and conversations that developed in conjunction with medical knowledge, however, did not divulge the sort of ideas Foucault elicited from other historical cases. In the early twentieth century, young readers were not expected to communicate their newly obtained sexual knowledge to others—only to behave decorously after a recitation of modest facts and sincere, if unelaborated, truisms. Communication was prophylactic, not confessional. Further, critics and historians have begun to raise questions about the applicability of Foucault's theories to the historical actualities of their domains.[10] While early twentieth-century print resources advised readers, broadly, about threats to their health and reproductive capabilities and urged premarital abstinence, any power embodied in these works was far from monolithic.[11]

Treatises for adolescents were challenged by individuals and government officials. Authors and publishers, far from exerting uncontentious influence, more often needed the credentials and credibility accumulated over the course of long careers to protect themselves against complaints. The distribution of sexual health texts for adolescent readers offers little evidence, then, of the mechanisms of scrutiny and power supposed by Foucauldian theory. Similarly, his questions about authorship, including the playfully ambiguous query "What difference does it make who is speaking?" seem alien to the reality that an individual's professional reputation, social prestige, and personal honor conferred respectability, even viability, upon controversial publishing endeavors.[12]

In considering how one might approach historical study, David M. Henkin has argued, "There is no reason why the study of the past needs to produce grand syntheses of eras or generalized claims. . . . Nonetheless, there are collective stories that can and should be told."[13] The development of sexual and reproductive health texts for adolescents at the turn of the twentieth century is one such episode. The transnational transmission of these texts testifies to mutual experiences of reading, acquiring knowledge, and negotiating cultural values. Students and other scholars who have listened to my presentations on these books and booklets sometimes share their personal experiences of this past. From students in Indiana to my colleague Jim Elmborg, who has the bookcases and the library that once belong to his Swedish grandfather, a shopkeeper and Lutheran minister who resettled in Kansas, their stories are much the same: a book published by Stall belonged to a family member, now deceased, and is in their possession. My research, then, seeks to account for how early twentieth-century hygiene texts wound up on all those shelves and in all those attics, waiting to be found by another generation.

Dr. Alfred Fournier, who instigated a professional meeting that he called the first International Conference for the Prevention of Syphilis and Venereal Diseases and subsequently founded the French Society for Sanitary and Moral Prophylaxis, was a significant force in ensuring adolescents' access to reproductive health information grounded in science. His research and reasoning about the problems represented by venereal disease motivated public information campaigns in France and abroad. Chapter 1, "French Origins of International Sexual Health Communication with Adolescents," places Fournier and his associations at the center of Progressive Era hygiene campaigns and defines his leadership. Beginning with his medical career in the late nineteenth century and extending to his eventual influence in French society, Fournier undertook a thorough, if philosophically conservative, examination of syphilis that resulted in his reputation, in the words of his contemporaries, as the leading syphilis expert of his generation. His role in creating the French Society for Sanitary and Moral Prophylaxis, its publications, and other texts indicates the centrality of his role to the nascent international effort to prevent sexually transmitted infection. The most serious consequence of these diseases, readers were warned, was sterility—a message that reflected real consequences of infection as well as contemporary French concerns about demographics. The Society's treatises were issued in multiple editions in France and translated abroad.

In addition to nonfiction booklets with authoritative interpretations of medical information as the basis for moral advice, warnings about the tragedy wrought by sexually transmitted infections were conveyed via the didactic drama *Les avariés,* which was translated into English as *Damaged Goods.* Chapter 2, "Initial Transnational Intersections: French Texts and American Culture," traces the relationships and the processes which made Fournier's work known to American audiences. The launch of the French Society for Sanitary and Moral Prophylaxis brought syphilis to the attention of the playwright Eugene Brieux, and *Les avariés,* a dramatization of the damage syphilis could do, was the result. Its translation into English followed a few years later, in collaboration with the reform-oriented dramatist George Bernard Shaw. Later, the Connecticut Society of Social Hygiene spurred further sales of the play. The subsequent novelization by Upton Sinclair is also noteworthy for its author's dialogues with French and English dramatists who made the play available, as well as the continued distribution of its message.

At the same time that these efforts played out, American physician Prince A. Morrow introduced his colleagues to the idea of a reform society with an informational mission. Although encouraged by self-motivated translations of his Society's texts, Fournier did not leave the distribution of health messages to chance and directed others to form societies like his in their home countries. Morrow's colleagues in the French Society for Sanitary and Moral Prophylaxis charged the New York physician with forming a parallel group in the United States. Ever dutiful, Morrow tried to interest American doctors in venereal disease prevention using diverse dimensions of the French Society's activism as a model for innovative communications with teens about reproductive health. He was among those who relied on Fournier's focus on literacy, scientific facts, and sensitivity to issues of gender and culture as the signature elements of an evolving effort.

Chapter 3, "*Social Hygiene vs. the Sexual Plagues* in Indiana and the World," further explains the means by which sexual and reproductive health information gained a presence in the United States and abroad. A common story about Morrow's recruiting of potential Society members is of the resulting, reluctant few who gathered in a New York City meeting room, but at least one man found Morrow's arguments serious and convincing. As secretary of public health for the state of Indiana, John N. Hurty waged an early and controversial campaign against the spread of syphilis, and his chief information product, *Social Hygiene vs. the Sexual Plagues,* was distributed nationally and internationally.

While Hurty formed a private group that supported his endeavor, *Social Hygiene vs. the Sexual Plagues* was published under the auspices of his state agency, and the partnership provided by the Indiana Society of Social Hygiene was acknowledged only to advocates who asked Hurty's advice about conducting this sort of campaign. Just as Hurty had learned from Morrow's encounter with the French reform group, others were interested in what Hurty accomplished, including international audiences. This outreach, however, did not impress Indiana government officials, who eventually compelled Hurty to discontinue the publication, a demand enforced by budgetary constraints. The state legislature's decision to curtail the distribution of sexual and reproductive health information was only one of the limitations publishers experienced in this era.

A prominent, prolific commercial author and publisher of hygiene literature also affected the availability of sexual and reproductive health information for audiences in the United States and abroad. Chapter 4, "What Young Readers Ought to Know: The Successful Selling of Sex Education," traces the popularity of books that melded religious ideology and reproductive health information, as indicated by the way these books were sold in the United States and around the world. These hardcover books excited sustained consumer interest. Their publisher, Sylvanus Stall, effectively created a significant print product and formed a global network of his own, but also owed much to the medical research and social reform promoted by Morrow and others. Titles in Stall's Self and Sex Series became lingering cultural icons, reflecting their durable position in the marketplace. Part of what made the Self and Sex Series sell was Stall's religion; his credentials as a minister and his connection with missionary groups protected his works with a propriety to which others could only aspire. His success and his attempts to expand his print empire prompted both imitators and complaints.

All who published in this period were obliged to defend the decency of their texts, reflective of real risks associated with producing sexual and reproductive health titles in the first decades of the twentieth century. Although hygiene authors corresponded and met with like-minded individuals and groups that supported their work, they nonetheless had to contend with sometimes unreceptive markets and government forces. The latter, particularly, infringed upon efforts to communicate the threats associated with unrestrained and unprotected intercourse, while the commercial viability of general audience titles by Stall had other consequences for the distribution of new work in this area. These tensions are discussed in Chapter 5, "Battling Books: Censorship, Conservatism, and Market Competition." Postal inspector Anthony Comstock, authorized by the eponymous Comstock Laws, disrupted networks that made reproductive health literature available to professional and public readers.

Comstock hindered publication and distribution of some materials, yet the decency of treatises was not the only legal issue that writers engaged. The moralistic language of prevention-oriented documents for the general public has become a significant scholarly theme, but a broad array of texts shows that Fournier and others still pursued knowledge of the best treatment options for sexually transmitted infection. These works were likewise translated and redistributed across national borders, albeit differently than before, as copyright protection became of increased interest once the viability of hygiene texts had been demonstrated. New scientific developments created new texts for purchase, rather than leading to substantive revision of earlier titles, whose circulation nonetheless continued.

However, when Winfield Scott Hall, a physician who taught at Northwestern University's medical school and published mainstream physiology texts in the latter years of the nineteenth century, turned his attention to adolescent sexual health in the twentieth century, he advanced arguments that other physicians and experts on adolescence had begun to reject as unscientific. His ever-more central position in public dialogues about social hygiene contrasted with his increasingly dated perspective on the medicine underlying his pronouncements about adolescent health. Hall's promotional strategies revealed his study of Stall's pioneering efforts and his emulation of others who developed innovative health texts for adolescents, but the medical man's enterprises never managed to outpace those of the minister. While implicitly upholding the integral role of literacy in maintaining health, a notion that was present at the start of this movement, later developments engaged the broader culture, rather than the culture of physicians and reformers.

Collectively, these works signal that despite scholarship that has understood Progressive Era sexual and reproductive health texts as a largely undifferentiated and moralistic literature, multiple motives grounded the production of these works. Similarities emerged because networks linked far-flung reformers, and cultural and legal phenomena demanded strategic approaches to authorship and publication. This information revolution, which saw the adolescent as a vulnerable individual who would benefit from recent scientific research, fostered a print culture that was both responsive and didactic, medically and morally concerned. By engaging sometimes disparate primary sources, this book articulates the avenues by which a wide-ranging group of reformers came to advocate reading as a means of ensuring health. Then as now, ideas about health and the body may become fixed on the page while maintaining greater fluidity in the laboratory and in clinical and social practice. A history of the processes and the people who rendered scientific findings into an extensive adolescent reading matter, then, must account for the limitations of medicine, the dynamics of culture, and the interests of commerce. Changing conditions both created and constrained an outpouring of print materials intended to shape a young person's sexuality.

These developments meant that the young reader, who once would have been fortunate to receive a thin booklet from a trusted doctor or a concerned family member was, within years, able to buy a text of his choosing from an unknown salesperson who asked only that the bill be paid. Until the spoken word, transmitted electronically, became debated as a new means of conveying health information, books were the means of battling venereal disease. Thus conditionally redeemed from their reputation as destroyers of health and enemies of morality, books about sex gained worldwide distribution. The course to this end was long, varied, and uneven. Authors' experiences as they endeavored to connect books and readers suggest the reason that John Hurty, in Indiana, had broached the subject of syphilis metaphorically rather than medically. By 1910, Hurty and many other distributors of reproductive health materials knew that fire posed dangers to any who sought to control it.

CHAPTER 1

FRENCH ORIGINS OF INTERNATIONAL SEXUAL HEALTH COMMUNICATION WITH ADOLESCENTS

The first questions which were posed were relative to youth.
Ought one enlighten students in the higher classes at teaching
centers? Ought one enlighten soldiers, sailors,
young people of the working classes? Alfred Fournier
presented the first response on these questions.

—JUSTIN SICARD DE PLAUZOLES

At the age of seventy, French physician Alfred Fournier turned, in the words of one colleague, his "prudent pen" to adolescents' risk for sexually transmitted infection.[1] The preeminent syphilologist of his generation, Fournier had become convinced that the secrecy and shame surrounding syphilis were conditions that allowed it to flourish.[2] It followed that communicating broadly, rather than only with other physicians, was essential to disease prevention. For years he had challenged cultural and professional norms that left the general public, particularly young people, ignorant and consequentially vulnerable to the long-term and even fatal consequences of sexually transmitted infection. His profound commitment, described as crusading by some contemporaries, culminated in his founding of a national association to serve this aim. This French anti–venereal disease society quickly grew to more than 300 members, and Fournier expected others to do the same sort of organizing whether they lived elsewhere in Europe or in the United States. His most renowned act, though, was the creation of the short treatise *Pour nos fils, quand ils auront 18 ans: quelques conseils d'un médecin,* first published in 1901. In *For Our Sons, When They Turn 18: Some Advice from a Doctor,* Fournier named the three known venereal diseases, depicted their consequences, and called upon young men to regard sexual experience as the reward of marriage rather than the prerogative of masculinity. Eventually this fifty-page booklet would find a broad readership and spark the creation of other health texts. Its existence, however, was possible only after the social and scientific developments of the recent past.

Around the middle of the nineteenth century, forces that would render germ theory a convincing explanation for illness coalesced, and individuals committed themselves to organizing for all sorts of social reform. Abolition, suffrage, and workers' rights were among the popular causes of the nineteenth century, while child welfare and eugenics would prevail in the next. Medicine and movements for the betterment of the human condition met, resulting in professional conferences that shared knowledge in hopes of preventing disease and human suffering. Significantly, these efforts were also intended to protect commercial interests and national vitality. First came meetings like the International Sanitary Conference of 1851, which focused on controlling the spread of cholera. This initial international collaboration was a novel endeavor whose recorded outcomes and disease containment strategies were shared only among participants.[3] From this first meeting in Paris, others would follow, directing attention to health threats whose significance was indicated by emergent scientific and technological developments. Before the end of the century, sexually transmitted infection became the object of this sort of international scrutiny and communication. The First International Congress of Dermatology and Syphiligraphy, held in Paris in 1889, was followed by two conferences dedicated to the prevention of syphilis and venereal disease in Brussels in 1899 and 1902.[4] Unlike the more limited 1851 meeting, the later international conferences hosted delegates from a diversity of nations. In addition to nearby European neighbors, physicians from Brazil, Denmark, the Congo, Iran, and Japan attended.[5]

At these meetings, physicians sought to repair the breach identified by writers like Dr. Homer Bostwick, who in 1848 claimed that European governments were considering how to respond to syphilis, while England and the United States left their citizens to suffer.[6] Half a century after Bostwick suggested that American doctors ought to emulate their European colleagues, the parties did meet to consider the common problem of preventing venereal disease, and the working group publicized its conclusions.[7] The gradual recognition that ignorance of reproductive health and its converse, venereal disease, were inherently dangerous in an era before effective cures led physicians, authors, and editors to present new audiences with medical facts. In 1902, doctors at the second Brussels conference created an education committee "which, inspired by existing brochures, shall serve as a means of instruction for the world in general."[8] This declaration transmitted Fournier's warnings to young men in other countries and resounded in later works like *Today's World Problem in Disease Prevention: A Non-Technical Discussion of Syphilis and Gonorrhea* by John Stokes of the Mayo Clinic. Such titles shared the aim of making what was once specialized medical knowledge comprehensible to readers who might have merely average educations. The new works designed to help young people avoid infection were part biology instruction and part conduct manual, typically complemented by measures of paternal advice and patriotic reverence. The project of writing about medicine for young readers created common ground, effectively reshaping the genre of popular health information by defying prevailing assumptions that the details of one's health would be discussed face-to-face, confidentially with a doctor, and that instruction in reproduction likewise occurred as a conversation between parent and child. Previously, much printed material that took sex as its subject was either a pretext for titillating content or a moralistic condemnation of anything other than married, procreative sex. An informative text that could be shared with a young woman who had recently taken her first job or a young man who had gone away to school would prove valuable, yet required its proponents to negotiate prevailing mores.

Reading in general, let alone turning the pages of a volume about sex, was not uniformly regarded as behavior to be encouraged in a young person. Authors of sexual health treatises confronted a long-held suspicion, described by Thomas Laqueur, which associated the reading individual and the deleterious practice of masturbation.[9] The fear that physical harm and moral degradation could result from reading, the belief that a book could exhibit seductive force, was exemplified by the eugenicist physician John H. Kellogg, who railed, "A bad book is as bad as an evil companion. In some respects it is even worse than a living teacher of vice, since it may cling to an individual at all times. It may follow him into the secrecy of his bed chamber. . . . A confirmed novel reader is almost as difficult to reform as a confirmed inebriate or opium-eater. . . . by reading of this kind, many are led to resort to self abuse for the gratification of passions which over-stimulation has made almost uncontrollable."[10] Even later writers who would have scoffed at Kellogg's high Victorian sensibilities warned that "books . . . have no small influence on adolescent sex ideals," singling out "the sentimental mush too easily available to unguided boys and girls" as a cause of "sexual disaster."[11] These attitudes led many writers to justify their decisions to write about sexuality, even when they did so from a medical perspective. Kellogg, who proclaimed his rationale self-evident with the rather caustic observation, "The publishers of this work offer no apology for presenting it to the reading public, since the wide prevalence of the evils which it exposes is sufficient warrant for publication," was an anomaly.[12] Fournier provided a model for those who wanted to assuage concerns that a stranger might infringe on a parent's responsibilities via the written word. He observed that young readers were in someone else's care but argued that new medical knowledge about disease demanded the introduction of scientific knowledge into discourse that had been idealized as domestic, familial, and personal. He praised conventional virtues such as modesty and propriety, while being among the first to make the case that awareness of syphilis and its dangers was not incongruent with the roles and the attitudes that well-brought-up young people should adopt. In time, the theme of protecting youth from unhealthy influences by demanding appropriate education would shape the work of the nascent child-study movement in America, too.

Scholarly characterizations of Victorian attitudes toward sexuality notwithstanding, the reform advocates who disseminated reproductive health treatises understood their work as a new and fundamentally sensitive enterprise.[13] By the first years of the twentieth century, professional experience and current medical literature encouraged reform-minded individuals to dismiss well-known titles as unsuitable. A small yet influential number of physicians deplored the enduring, voyeuristic appeal of the popular marriage manual *Aristotle's Masterpiece*, and even the more staid *Plain Facts for Old and Young: Embracing the Natural History and Hygiene of Organic Life* by Kellogg. While undoubtedly aware of these and other texts bearing out Roy Porter and Lesley Hall's observation that "print culture brought sex books into prominence," the men who united to promote reproductive health characterized their concerns as grounded in medicine, morality, and futurity.[14] In their deliberations, Fournier and his colleagues reviewed extant sources and concluded, "A book responding to these multiple exigencies does not exist, at least to our knowledge."[15]

Popularizing authoritative information without the risqué elements with which some writers had enlivened this genre was central to their aims of repairing general ignorance and misinformation. Two lacunae were evident: the adolescent as the intended reader and the subject of disease, scientifically treated. Helen Lefkowitz Horowitz has evaluated the Victorian-era reading of works like *Aristotle's Masterpiece,* noting both this book's explicit conjugal content and the outrage that resulted when unmarried adolescents were found consulting it.[16] Porter and Hall, too, have commented on lingering attitudes toward the youthful readership of manuals and treatises that took sex as their subject: "Such individuals had no legitimate business having a sex life at all; was it not, therefore, needlessly provocative to put in their hands the very means for finding out about forbidden practices?"[17] Early twentieth-century medical reformers who wanted the public to consider the evolving research on sexually transmitted infection would confront questions and attitudes that had changed little since the eighteenth century.[18] These older perspectives, which wore the guise of common knowledge, also dismissed the seriousness of venereal disease.

To demonstrate that venereal disease in general and syphilis in particular posed real threats to well-being, reformers first had to persuade practitioners and the public that long-held assumptions about health were fundamentally mistaken. When Fournier presented his rationale for discussing sex with adolescents to an international audience, the medical profession was still studying the diseases he warned against, debating the appropriate clinical response to them. He contended, in his early activism, that not only was syphilis far more virulent than believed, and thus more damaging than previously thought, but that gonorrhea, once regarded as little more than a symptom of a young man's sexual initiation, had serious consequences, too.

Before Fournier could do more than aid individual patients who arrived at his clinic lamenting their ignorance with cries of "I am lost!" and "I didn't know," he had to ensure that future doctors received accurate information about sexually transmitted infection in their preparation for practice.[19] As one of his colleagues recalled in a tribute to the noted physician's accomplishments, Fournier changed medical education, which had previously relegated syphilis to the status of a minor ailment.[20] He persuaded physicians that neither condition was an insignificant one that should simply be allowed to run its course. "*Laisser aller* means nothing else but harm to the patient: that is my firm conviction," Fournier wrote.[21] He counseled, "Syphilis, in fact, is not what it generally appears. In reality, it's something else entirely. It's an unyielding infection, permanent, ultra-fecund in all its manifestations, some of them slight, others important and more serious, some of them even fatal. In reality it's a disastrous malady, baneful, because of the multiple dangers that it carries: danger to the individual, danger that may be hereditary, and we add also, danger to society."[22] Not all were immediately receptive to his message.

Instead, they clung to doubts made tenable by the scarcity of reliable information about syphilis and other sexually transmitted infections, a void revealed in multiple facets of late nineteenth- and early twentieth-century medical literature. For the most incisive perspective, medical men looked to experts working in continental European cities. Among these figures was Philippe Ricord, who in 1838 had proved that gonorrhea and syphilis were in fact two distinct diseases, the latter with profoundly serious consequences. The words of another contemporary physician, whose accolades envisioned the Frenchman with a nearly godlike power, signaled the contemporary importance of Ricord's work: "M. Ricord has reduced to order that which before was wholly devoid of system. Light has broken in upon the darkness of ignorance and superstition, and henceforth we may hope to see the pathology of syphilis assume that rank, which, by reason of the universal prevalence of the disease, and of its grave consequences on the afflicted individual and on succeeding generations, it so well deserves."[23] Ricord led the transition to research that identified venereal diseases as serious threats to health. Regardless of the acclaim and eventual recognition of the value of Ricord's core finding, his contentions about the treatment of syphilis would be revised by Fournier, who, by chance, had become his student.

While hailing Ricord's clarification of their understanding of venereal disease, his peers recognized persistent difficulties in treatment and even in accounting for how many cases there might be. No longer content with maxims that concluded simply, "the higher the degree of civilization, the greater the prevalence of syphilis," they began to estimate infection rates based on the number of individuals treated in city hospitals or clinics.[24] Frustrated by the admitted limitations of their methods, doctors and public health officials would later label the disease "the despair of statisticians" and a "statistical anarchy."[25] By the turn of the century, many agreed that the disease was far too prevalent, that its effects were lasting, and that it must be prevented.

The shortcomings of professional knowledge impeded prevention goals for some time, even as advances began to accumulate. Experts' specializations, typically in dermatology, reflected real limitations in what was known about venereal diseases by responding to their manifestations as sores and skin discolorations. Both the connection and the incipient differentiation between syphilis and unrelated skin conditions can be seen in practitioners' reference manuals of the late nineteenth century. One, *A Clinical Atlas of Venereal and Skin Diseases Including Diagnosis, Prognosis & Treatment*, was a massive volume that aided treatment by depicting, in full-color illustrations, the characteristic skin conditions symptomatic of syphilis.[26]

Another physician-author noted the reconsideration-in-progress with a decided, if considered, skepticism: "One is forcibly impressed with the view that syphilis . . . is a disease of microbic origin; but, striking as is the probability, the facts in our possession to-day do not warrant us to go as far as some authors who unhesitatingly argue syphilis is a disease of bacterial origin." One ought not accept that a micro-organism caused syphilis because of the imprecise nature of the evidence, the author indicated, continuing, "A number of observers have found in active and early syphilitic lesions certain micro-organisms which have been revealed by delicate staining methods, but their numbers have been small, their presence not absolutely constant, and, furthermore, no cultures have been made."[27]

Such doubts were unexceptional, and disbelievers were not always so scientifically dispassionate. A full two decades following Fournier's call for activism, Stokes lamented that too many of his colleagues still failed to respond to venereal disease as a treatable health condition rather than a sign of disgrace. He criticized the public and the profession alike: "Even highly trained, cultivated and well-informed people, not excluding from that number physicians of wide experience, still cherish the lingering belief that syphilis is largely, and gonorrhea almost exclusively, a proof of moral degradation and the property of down and outs."[28] In other words, physicians still relied on the conclusions of an older medical literature that had not moved beyond a tenuous and groping effort to define an adverse health condition whose causes were not yet identifiable.

The source of sexually transmitted infections was often characterized, in the chronologies that attempted to explain its ominous presence in the modern city, as having its origins elsewhere, as being caused by people at some remove from the writer and his surroundings. Germ theory did not make immediate inroads into accounts of disease transmission. Turn-of-the-century authors offered etiologies of syphilis in which its affliction of Europe was linked either to fifteenth-century explorations of the Americas or to the aftermath of military invasions of European nations during the wars of this same period. One nation had syphilis and visited it upon another, typically through military or colonial aggression. Thus, in 1860, when Fournier advanced the distinctive argument that "syphilis always begins with a particular ailment, the chancre," he was responding to a common authorial practice, which traced the ailment not to the patient's body, but to someone else's.[29] Nationally derived epithets for syphilis—in which the British referred to the ailment as the French pox, and the French in turn attributed it to the Italians—continued this pattern. This gave rise to naming a person or a place as diseased without considering how or why infection prevailed, a tendency that continued in Progressive Era reform literature that warned men away from prostitutes.

The prostitute's certain depravity was condemned more often than it was analyzed for any meaningful resolution of her presumed health and economic problems.[30] The fallen and infected woman's state figured in both medical accounts of disease and literary forms that took up the prevention theme, notably in the role of an embittered, nearly deranged woman who knowingly infected others to revenge her own misery. In these accounts, prostitutes were morally and physically corrupted. Even after physicians became less concerned with the disease's remote origins, beliefs about its contemporary sites still impeded diagnosis and treatment.

Doctors who wrote for other doctors had for some time promoted the idea that men contracted syphilis in the city. The scenario was envisioned this way: "A stranger in the city sometimes loses his watch or pocket book at what are called panel houses. He goes to the police-office, the officers are set on the track, the offenders are arrested, and sometimes the property recovered, and the thieves are sent to prison. But a countryman may be robbed of health, happiness, and life itself, without any such remedy, or any remedy other than a prompt application for medical advice, and then it is an even chance if he does not fall into the hands of quackery."[31] Fournier, however, located syphilis and gonorrhea in the countryside as well as the city, contradicting pastoral assumptions that contrasted healthy rural living with urban blight and infection. His earliest American colleagues also warned of "neglected cases" that were overlooked because they occurred where they were not anticipated, whether in a rural environment or a presumably virtuous young woman. This problem, the so-called innocent infection, referred to the wife infected because of her husband's philandering, the victim of the social kiss or the shared cup at a public rest stop, or the infant who contracted his parents' disease.[32] The exculpatory language developed to communicate with the public implied sexually transmitted infection could be acquired blamelessly, and American physician L. Duncan Bulkley challenged his colleagues to understand that "syphilis is to be looked for and expected under any circumstance of life, and no purity of character or correctness of living insures against the possibility of acquiring the disease."[33] The geography of the disease and the effort of locating infected bodies seemed to befuddle practitioners only recently convinced that they ought to treat it at all

Thus, at the start of the twentieth century, physicians saw syphilis as an "insidious disease" which, "though nothing like so fatal as tuberculosis, is nearly as widespread, and a vast amount of ill health and misery result from it."[34] The latter disease, itself referred to as the white plague, became an analogy to explain the dangers of the former, and as with so many other aspects of the effort to communicate with the public, Fournier's writings contain one of the earliest uses of this simile.[35] Difficulties of diagnosis and treatment resulted, in part, from reliance on symptoms to indicate the disease's presence or supposed cure. When prominent United States physicians, many of whom served as delegates to the 1899 International Conference for the Prevention of Syphilis and Venereal Disease held in Brussels, shortly afterward tried to make state-of-the-art knowledge available to other American physicians, the microbe that caused syphilis had not yet been identified. That discovery, of the *spirochaeta pallida* by Schaudinn and Hoffman, took place a few years later, in 1905. The Wasserman test, which detected the recently discovered source, followed in 1906; interpreting its results, however, remained notoriously imprecise. As physicians' understanding of the limitations of their abilities to cure diseases like syphilis grew, their commitment to prevention increased.

Prevention was inherently linked, in this era, to sexual restraint, and the coupling of health and abstinence required doctors to debunk any number of myths about sex. Fournier succinctly urged monogamy: "The sole means of avoiding syphilis is chastity before marriage. . . . For husbands there is no other means of avoiding syphilis than conjugal fidelity."[36] In this statement, he quietly sidestepped both female desire and what physicians dubbed "the sexual necessity," a lingering scientific conviction that semen not regularly expelled from the male body would decay within, metamorphosing from procreative germ to noxious substance. Paul Marrin went so far as to claim that the hazards of male celibacy extended to criminal behavior and suicide.[37] The case for celibacy required persuasion, and testimonials to the way male vigor and health served the weaker sex by protecting women from physical or moral endangerment attempted to assure male recipients of these new health messages that masculinity had other expressions besides sexuality.

Fournier was one of few writers who did not discuss masturbation, which disquieted many reformers even before physicians attempted to dissuade young men from casual sex. Ordinarily authors warned against the practice, telling young people that the sins of the flesh would manifest themselves as readily recognizable conditions; the telltale signs included everything from lethargy and acne to insanity. The standing scientific evidence for these harms was refuted early in the twentieth century, but fearmongering messages could still be found on the pages of hygiene treatises decades later. That masturbation offended older sensibilities but posed no threat to well-being was seldom openly acknowledged. Collectively, these works encouraged reproductive sex, a capacity preserved through self-control, and frowned upon any sort of corporeal indulgence. Even foods thought to foster the passions, through spices and strong flavors, were discouraged.

Thus, innovations in medical knowledge and technology, coupled with reform impulses, eventually yielded print materials that warned young people about the consequences of venereal disease. At the same time that physicians saw the dynamic and quickening elements of modernity, like transportation and urban employment, as factors that increased the risk of disease, they also relied on emerging technologies in the interest of prevention. New hot-metal type increased the ease and decreased the costs of printing conference proceedings and tracts that recorded the evidence for hygienic claims. It was not uncommon for producers of health titles to consider the look and feel of the works they created, assessing the impression that material aspects of book design and printing would have on a young reader. As works about sexual health distanced themselves from their dubious nineteenth-century predecessors, texts achieved the status of prophylactics against disease, even among writers with rather conservative sensibilities.

The twentieth-century distribution of hygiene texts that originated in France was a definitive element of a transnational prevention movement. Claude Quétel has voiced skepticism about the immediate effect of these informational campaigns, and it has been argued that only after 1910, particularly in the years proximate to World War I, did nations confront the problem of venereal disease.[38] This argument is given credence by scholarship that focuses on health campaigns for military men and on the subsequent development of school-based hygiene programs for children. Yet the roots of serious, sustained prevention efforts were developed prior to official governmental campaigns, and their efficacy is signaled by the transnational dissemination of texts resulting from these early endeavors, as well as the way their messages later resurfaced. Like the earlier activity focused on cholera, this effort began in France, instigated by a prominent doctor and instructor who believed that scientific knowledge required physicians to communicate the threat of sexually transmitted infection. Eventually, those who followed in his footsteps included other physicians and reformers, writers and editors, even dramatists and novelists. Collectively, their texts transformed knowledge that was once the technical, professional substance of medicine into reading matter for adolescents in countries throughout the world.

The Far-Reaching Work of the French Society for Sanitary and Moral Prophylaxis

In late nineteenth-century Paris, Fournier enjoyed some renown, and in the late twentieth century, physicians highlighted the lasting significance of his work and the singularity of his personality.[39] His fellow physicians credited him with a brilliant career while still a student, describing him as an incisive translator of Latin texts who linked current medical problems to their classical origins and, in all he wrote, a first-rate stylist.[40] After studying with Ricord, he went on to revise his instructor's long-standing explanations of syphilitic transmission and to demonstrate that the disease caused paralysis and dementia.[41]

Fournier's publication of his notes on Ricord's lectures in 1860, though, was among the younger physician's early writing endeavors.[42] A subsequent essay for the *Dictionnaire de Jaccoud* outlined the effects of alcoholism, arguing that the condition aggravated ailments like syphilis.[43] Near the turn of the century he had become a leading French physician, seeing patients and training new doctors at the prestigious, specialized Hôpital St-Louis in Paris. By this time, it was believed that as many as one in seven of his countrymen were infected with syphilis.[44] His ensuing texts on venereal disease were hailed as "the classics of modern syphilography," and his instruction of medical students was regarded with acclaim because of the innovative knowledge he shared.[45] His skill was attributed to innate intelligence and a precise memory, as well as a facility with language. In a preface to his research, Fournier once asked, "May I hope, then, that the difficulties of this work will also gain me the indulgence of my listeners?"[46] Despite British feminist Josephine Butler's objections to his views on prostitution, medical audiences readily assented to his propositions about the problems that resulted from venereal disease. One colleague said that in his half-century of teaching, "Fournier contributed powerfully to dispelling our ignorance."[47]

As a physician and a faculty member, Fournier circulated among France's elite, yet also had contact with those who were less privileged; each group influenced his thinking and formed an audience for his ideas about disease prevention. Baron Henri de Rothschild recalled him as one of the men his mother selected to educate him, someone who sought to guide his personal and professional conduct. The young nobleman, as a medical student, could not evade Fournier's awareness of his private life or his comments about its implications for his eventual marriage.[48] This observation of individuals' lives, their relationships and their risks, was integral to Fournier's knowledge of the nature of syphilis and of the broad ignorance surrounding it. Personalized understanding also came about through Fournier's contact with patients in the medical practice that he maintained in addition to his professorship.[49] The senior physician recorded data from clinical consultations that showed, convincingly, the contagiousness of syphilis in its later stages. His reputation as a learned and compassionate doctor, in turn, ensured a "considerable clientele."[50]

Fournier was among the first to shift attention from professional dialogues about the possibilities of inoculation to a more open communication about prevention, and his individual interactions transformed into a broader agenda. He was credited with conceptualizing sexually transmitted infection as social disease or one whose effects extended beyond the individual to the family and even society.[51] The phenomenon of social disease entailed certain duties: the physician was obligated to counsel the public about prevention, and the individual, in Fournier's thinking, was bound to restrain his sexual impulses in the interest of health. Although the phrase and these sentiments would be criticized by later physicians who argued that this sort of rhetoric opened the way for moralistic opposition to sound medicine, many of his contemporaries found it a compelling explanation for the seriousness of venereal disease. His colleagues complimented his clarity and elegance of expression, noting that its persuasive and expert tenor added power to his convictions.[52]

Significantly, Fournier did not restrict his perspective on health to questions that could be resolved by scientific study. The sentiment that disease punished the guilty was pervasive, if not within the profession then in society at large, and this attitude was one that he sought to overturn.[53] Even the guilty suffered, Fournier argued, and that suffering should be relieved by contemporary medicine.

He saw romantic attraction and physical well-being as inextricably linked. Medical advice about the risks sex involved had to deal as frankly with feelings as it did with infection, Fournier contended, and for this he turned to the classical figures involved in his first academic recognition. One colleague recalled, "Fournier consecrated his life to the study of syphilis and its dangers, as this abominable evil is intimately bound to the physiology of love. . . . It would be difficult not to talk about Venus when we treat venereal disease."[54] Fournier's decidedly unscientific musings on the matter were remembered thus: "Everything conspires to provoke desire: women's coquetry, art, literature, poetry. . . . Poets consecrate their most beautiful songs to love, considering it even a professional necessity. . . . Why so many difficulties in the practice of virtue? It's that Venus is mistress of the world."[55] As well as the personification of love and sexual desire, women were wives and mothers, as Fournier understood them. His ideas about women could be somewhat conservative, despite his wish to liberate people from long-held misperceptions about venereal disease. That the prominent doctor's expansive views were tempered with this sort of moderation led his colleagues to see him as erudite, accomplished, and gentlemanly.

These traits enabled him to advocate for reform, over the course of years, in professional and government circles. When the French Academy of Medicine sought authoritative responses to a committee report issued in 1887, Fournier was among the experts called upon for testi-

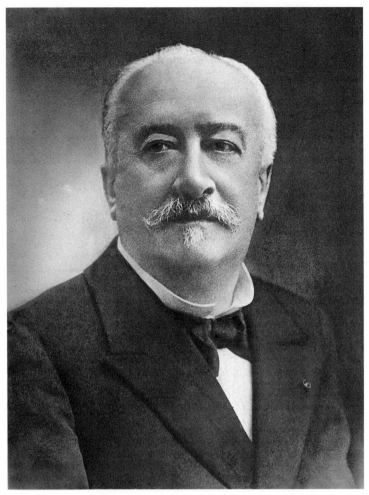

1. This undated photograph of Alfred Fournier shows him as he would have appeared to colleagues and patients during the years in which he advocated for informing the general public, and adolescents in particular, about venereal disease. Wellcome Library, London. Reproduced with permission.

mony about declining birth rates. He ably and persuasively explained the causal role of syphilis in disability, stillbirths, and sterility, and the Academy's endorsement of his argument was unanimous.[56] To Fournier, the implications of his data were clear: if a sexually transmitted infection could not be cured, it could only be prevented. This meant that all adolescents must be given information about health risks and reproduction before they became sexually active. His analysis provided a rationale for disease prevention, sanctioned by his peers and acknowledged by many in government.

As someone with knowledge and reputation, Fournier sought to influence leaders who could institute new policies, and in turn, bring about changes that would decrease the incidence of disease. Crucially, his professional opinions were sufficiently persuasive to bring many to believe in the importance of a fundamental change in public understanding of reproductive health; his proposition, however, that the French government itself should carry out this effort was not accepted. Though still controversial, his expertise and his interpretation of a perceived threat to the French state made the rather radical case for sex education credible. Unable to bring about a government program for public education in reproductive health, Fournier formed an organization, whose membership was primarily medical men like himself, to take up the cause. Years of advocacy preceded his founding, in the spring of 1901, the French Society for Sanitary and Moral Prophylaxis (SFPSM).[57]

The Society's name resulted from perceptions that a league against syphilis, as Fournier would have preferred, was simply too contentious.[58] While retaining conventional ideals of virtue, the Society sought to encourage new values with regard to personal and public health that aligned its work, philosophically, with the ebb of natalist campaigns that had emerged in the nineteenth century. Membership was open to any individual who paid annual dues of ten francs, provided two current members would "guarantee the honor of the candidate."[59] Far more men than women became members, and many physicians joined, but a range of professions were represented on the Society's rosters. Judith Surkis has observed, "Notable members were luminaries in the fields of law and administration, as well as politics."[60] A monthly bulletin recorded their discussions. This publication itself carried out a central element of the Society's twofold mission, "the study of all proper means of putting its concerns in writing to diminish the frequency of venereal disease, particularly syphilis."[61] In its declaration of purpose and identity, Fournier's Society linked literacy and disease prevention. To convey this new morality of health, which insisted on knowledge of sex and the body derived from recent medical research, Fournier instigated the publication of two booklets advising young people about the existence of and potential harm posed by sexually transmitted infections.

The first of the forty-plus-page brochures was introduced shortly after the Society's inception, and few copies from the first printing survive. In addition to preliminary versions reproduced in the Society's bulletin, the second edition of *For Our Sons, When They Turn 18: Some Advice from a Doctor* and the third revision of *For Our Daughters, When Their Mothers Judge This Advice Necessary*, both printed in 1905, remain to document an early twentieth-century mix of medical and social messages intended to warn French teens of the consequences of failing to protect their sexual and reproductive health. Fournier wrote the pamphlet for male readers, *Pour nos fils,* and Dr. Charles Burlureaux, another a member of the Society, authored the companion pamphlet for young women, eventually titled *Pour nos filles.* (An earlier edition of the latter bore the rather sensational title *Le peril venerien, conseils aux jeune filles* as the result of a ballot of possible titles.[62] The renaming of this work was only one dimension of the association's continuing communication with female readers, which was renewed in the 1920s under the auspices of a Committee for Female Education, formed in conjunction with the government's Ministry of Health.[63]) Current medical research and cultural norms alike were invoked in the Society's innovative treatises. These works addressed young people's developing sexuality and appealed to their future as French parents, advising male and female readers that pre-marital abstinence and monogamous marriage were the only sureties against a sexually transmitted infection that could deny them the possibility of bearing healthy children.

A strategic yet nonetheless, to some contemporary eyes, startling departure from conventions that considered information about sex the province of married individuals and medical men, these texts became widely influential beyond their immediate audience. Translations of the explanations that Fournier and his colleagues made to French adolescents reached readers in Europe, Indonesia, and the Americas during the next two decades. In this, the publications of the French Society for Sanitary and Moral Prophylaxis constituted the origins of a global effort to prevent sexually transmitted infection through outreach to young adults, creating both the first mass readership of sexual and reproductive health information and a continuing series of international conversations among physicians and reformers about health, sexuality, and adolescence. These pamphlets represented a considered and influential effort to engage young people as an audience for rapidly changing knowledge in health science.

Fournier's Adolescent Readers

Understanding the adolescent as an individual at the threshold of adulthood, yet different from both younger children and older adults, was at the core of Fournier's thinking about disease prevention. He and his colleagues recognized the importance of reaching young people during this developmental stage, once early youth had passed, but before teenagers became sexually active. This phase, as Fournier and other physicians understood it, represented a nexus of social, emotional, and physical transitions. Maturation was considered comprehensively in the Society's communications, reflecting contemporary awareness of the potential and the vulnerabilities inherent in this time of life.[64] In addition to defining reproduction as an aspect of public health, Fournier asked his colleagues to see the readers of these pamphlets as having entered a liminal period distinct from true adulthood. While the young men and women in whom the Society took interest seemed much like adults, capable of acting like them in many ways, sexuality was new to them, and they were still developing intellectually and morally. In framing his readership in these terms, Fournier joined in conversation with another profession.

It has been argued that American psychologist G. Stanley Hall invented the concept of adolescence in the early twentieth century, imbuing it with a sexuality that has since become its defining feature.[65] Once a student of William James's at Harvard, Hall became a professor and was later named president of Clark University. His credits are

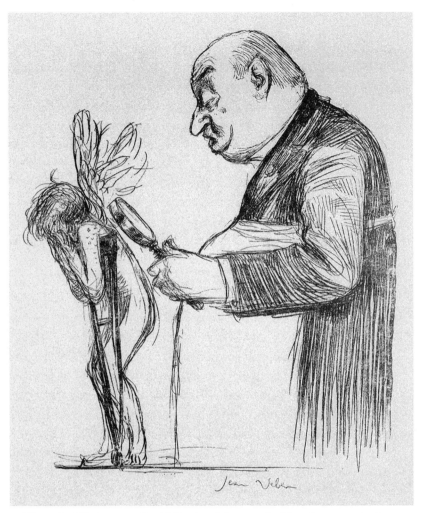

2. "Fournier Ministers to Cupid," a sketch by popular French cartoonist Jean Veber. Wellcome Library, London. Reproduced with permission.

numerous, revealing both his importance and his energetic commitment to the field: Hall created the first psychology laboratory, taught several individuals who subsequently became prominent psychologists, and was a founder of journals and the American Psychological Association. His views were influential in the academy and in the larger culture. Of all his efforts, though, his focus on the adolescent, whom he regarded as particularly susceptible to vice and the challenges of modernity, most captured the popular imagination. Even his chief critic, Columbia University biology professor Maurice Bigelow, acknowledged Hall's role in directing sustained attention to adolescence in American culture.[66]

In the two-volume survey of *Adolescence,* Hall attempted to describe comprehensively the condition of young people: their physical, mental, and emotional growth; their sexual and reproductive capabilities; their presence in the criminal system; and the way they were represented in literature.[67] His pronouncements, elaborated over the course of more than 1,000 pages published in 1904, would echo in the perspectives of his contemporaries and those of later writers as well. A reviewer for *The Dial* called the work "monumental" in recognition of its size and its standing.[68] A critical few, among them Bigelow and E. L. Thorndike, who rather brazenly lambasted *Adolescence* as "chock full of errors, masturbation, and Jesus," would contest Hall's conclusions as unscientific; however, reformers like physician Prince A. Morrow relied on this distinctive view of adolescence to justify sexual health education.[69] Given Bigelow's eventual leadership role in the American Social Health Association, which grew out of Morrow's efforts to form an association like Fournier's in New York, Morrow's preference for the way Hall explained adolescence attests strikingly to the power this perspective had in the medical community. The voices raised against Hall never seriously contested his authority, and for decades his commentaries on the problems of adolescence inspired others to share his concerns.

Not only was this phase inherently difficult, Hall argued, twentieth-century adolescence was more fraught with risk than ever before. "Modern life is hard, and in many respects increasingly so, on youth," he wrote.[70] He remembered a halcyon past when the transition to adulthood was simpler and contended that American social support for young people's maturation was inadequate. Like others dismayed by the anonymity and the press of economically important urban centers, he contended that a young person was unprepared to cope with the strains of employment and the ever-present temptations of city life. Society's "mad rush for sudden wealth and the reckless fashions set by its gilded youth" created issues that he enumerated in hopes of redress.[71] Among the problems young people encountered, Hall recognized conditions that would become Progressive Era causes: he was dismayed at the nature of "our urbanized hothouse life" and warned that sex wreaked "havoc in the form of secret vice, debauch, disease and enfeebled heredity."[72] His perception of adolescence, then, was not simply sexualized; it was also intrinsically eugenic, and his scrutiny of adolescence, like that of so many reformers of this era, revolved around notions of race, health, and reproduction. This focus also reflected Hall's reliance on ideas circulating in the medical community, whose international literature he cited in his massive two-volume work. Like many other activists of the time, he was concerned with ensuring normal, healthy development. Adolescent psychology, as it originated under Hall, was about understanding forces that might cause turmoil, in order to guide young people safely to a rational, productive adulthood.

Adolescence was universal, but its demands of each sex differed. Its onset was sudden, he declared, in sharp contrast with Bigelow's gradual development thesis.[73] He constructed a framework of adolescence that codified fundamental and biologically driven differences between the sexes, the first signs of which appeared by age 12. Hall's conviction that, at this age, a girl "divines, discriminates, and the male acts, does, and learns by doing" was reported to members of the American medical profession, who responded favorably.[74] He described young women's adolescence as centered on "establishing a normal periodicity to which all else must be subsumed, her preparation for maternity." Young men, he believed, were properly made vigorous and valiant by a rightly directed preparation for adult roles as husband and father. Young people confronted profound difficulties as they experienced these dramatic internal changes, and the result was a time of "storm and stress." Exchanging youthful consciousness for a more mature perspective, signaled by the acceptance of attitudes conducive to upholding the values of society and family, was essentially "a new birth."[75]

Hall hoped young people would acquire ideals conducive to maintaining a stable society, and he linked mental preparation for adult life with bodily condition, which allied him with many in medicine. He explained that teens could be encouraged toward adulthood by channeling their behavior in suitably gendered ways, an idea that he arrived at after consulting innumerable writers and researchers. Male adolescents were to partake in structured activities, females were advised to follow a passive regime, and defying these prescriptions was shown to lead to ruin or, in any case, childlessness. While Hall counseled young men to release an enduring, primitive urge to fight through rule-governed wrestling and boxing matches, he insisted that it was necessary that female adolescents avoid intellectual strain to ensure their capacity for child-bearing. For all he deplored masturbation, he was among those who regarded it as a self-indulgent depletion of vitality rather than a self-destructive path to madness. Heterosexuality was presumed; homosexuality was the result of inappropriate conditions for physical and spiritual growth.

To justify these pronouncements, Hall referred to sources as many and varied as Aristotle and the lives of the saints, the Shattuck Lecture in Massachusetts, and the publications of late nineteenth-century German and Italian psychologists. He drew on a range of research material, from embryonic dissection studies to surveys of soldiers, priests, and prostitutes that endeavored to understand the part masturbation played in adolescent development (his reaction to these research reports, which found overwhelmingly that it was a common practice, was to cast doubt on sampling and other issues of methodology).[76] Hall challenged writers who voiced pessimism about future generations; instead, he held that it was the earnest strivings of adolescents against vice and self-indulgence that created the prospect of a better society.[77] Fournier himself was among the experts whose studies of young people's development and health contributed to Hall's work.

It is unsurprising, then, that the idea of the adolescent as an individual whose life was changed by the development of sexual impulses and challenged by the conditions of modern living was clearly present in the writings of Fournier and his SFPSM colleagues. They regarded adolescents as individuals in transition, "no longer children" as Fournier told his young male audience, experiencing feelings that would "awaken progressively." "A new preoccupation takes hold of you," Fournier wrote. "One aspiration rouses you; pure or impure, one desire incites you. Let us speak cleanly: woman is born for you."[78]

While Burlureaux did not envision that his female readers would feel the stirrings of sexuality in quite this way, an early version of *Pour nos filles* circulated among SFPSM members recognized that young women were excited about romance and curious about what it meant to fall in love. Initially and in significant contrast to other reformers who worried that thoughts of love could turn a young woman's fancy where it ought not go, Burlureaux refused to reproach young women who dreamed of love. Instead and not unlike Fournier's earlier paean to Venus, his colleague's first account of female maturation saw love as the prime mover of the adolescent years. Burlureaux intended to tell young women that love was "the aim of life" and "the leading word on your lips, a word dear to young women above all others, a word that envelopes you with its gentle vibrations, like a caress."[79] Such suggestive images were omitted from the text that was ultimately distributed to the public. Rather than proclaiming that one's inclination to love and romance was natural and God-given, as Burlureaux had in this early version, the final form described an innocent moment when young women exchanged a fondness for dolls for envy of their recently married friends' children or, more darkly, became susceptible to the attractions of a romantic hero in the pages of a novel.[80]

His colleagues responded to his vision of sensual female adolescence with insistence that readers be warned about the disgrace of seduction and this only through the mediation of their mothers.[81] Adolphe Pinard, the physician who advanced *puericulture*, a eugenic theory of early infant care, expressed doubts about the enterprise, cautioning, "The time has not come to give such instruction to young girls, no more the working classes than the *bourgeoises*."[82] Pinard's doubts, in light of his status as a celebrated physician and his advocacy for a manual explaining venereal disease to the newly married, were powerful counters to Burlureaux's liberal text.[83] These voices altered Burlureaux's ambitious, even revolutionary, ideas. While young men became lustful in adolescence, young women desired only motherhood, at least in the chaste print of health texts.

Both pamphlets, though, characterized adolescence as a time of change, when sexual attraction and reproduction became newly important. In these texts and the discussions surrounding them, members of the SFPSM, while somewhat short of the depth of interest demonstrated by Hall, recognized that young people went through a developmental phase between their lives as children in their parents' households and the time when they would, according to the expectations of anxious French demographers, bear their own children.[84] Like Hall, and yet differently, the Society saw adolescents as the foundation of an improved society.

One of Fournier's medical colleagues remembered adolescents as the Society's immediate concern: "The first questions which were posed were relative to youth. Ought one to enlighten students in the higher classes at teaching centers? Ought one to enlighten soldiers, sailors, young people of the working classes? Alfred Fournier presented the first response on these questions."[85] Fournier's strong convictions resulted in some of the earliest science-based writings about sex and health for unmarried, teenaged readers. Although these texts were hardly free of contemporary ideologies of sex, class, and gender, their authors regarded young people as individuals whose physical and moral well-being would be safeguarded by knowledge only recently derived from medical research. Even among proponents of young people's education, the proposition of sharing so much information was hotly debated.[86] The point of view put forth by one Society member during a meeting over the proposed publication was not universally shared: "There is a world of difference between ignorance and innocence, between modesty and prudery. The most chaste ears may hear what we would say to them: new wives, even virgins, may, without impropriety, see and read that which we want to put before their eyes."[87] From this controversial perspective, innocence lay in modest conduct rather than in ignorance of reproductive matters, which subsequent hygiene reformers would articulate in the slogan "Innocence not ignorance" as the ideal to be encouraged in adolescents.[88]

The primary audience for these brochures was, according to their titles, adolescents, but Fournier and the Society's membership believed that parents must be involved in children's education. Deliberation of the *Filles* publication directly acknowledged parents' roles in guiding their daughters, as well as divisions within the Society over the question of female education. In introducing Burlureaux's text, Fournier indicated the propriety of familial protection for young female readers, as well as his respect for such conventions:

It is such advice that a mother—and *a fortiori,* a father—can be made to feel uncertain in giving to her daughter; also, it is these kinds of advice that a doctor has the sole competence to formulate, but he does not have the liberty of addressing a young woman without the assent of her family. So, mothers of families and especially of young working women, read these pages; and if, as we hope, you find them proper to instruct and protect your daughters against the many dangers that may menace them, allow them to read from this little work, which has only their safeguard as its intention.[89]

This preface suggests that Jill Harsin's complaint against Fournier as someone who "fully advocated the conventional practices that left women at risk" is overstated, revealing instead the ways in which the Society confronted the norms of early twentieth-century French culture.[90] While Burlureaux lamented the broad reluctance to allow female teens access to information about reproductive health, he conceded that the Society could not provide instruction to adolescent girls without their parents' assent.[91] Throughout *Pour nos filles,* he deferred to the ideal of the female audience as protected while young and then, once a mother, an informed protector herself.

Safeguards, however, were not only for young women. Male readers, too, were regarded as benefiting from parental attention. Fournier envisioned himself encountering a father to whom he could present *For Our Sons,* who would share it with his child. "I don't want to leave you without giving you, for your son, a little brochure which may be useful to him. Read it first, then, if you judge it appropriate, give it to him on my behalf, and then let us talk!" Fournier urged the imagined parent.[92] Neither male nor female readers, then, were intended to receive these booklets without familial consent.

This way of thinking about adolescence relies on features beyond those found in the professional literature, such as transition and sexuality; it also envisions the adolescent of either sex as a reader, an idea Fournier developed within his own family circle. Although Sirkus derided Fournier for having "posed as a father and as an ally of fathers," Fournier in fact had a lively, loving family, including a son who joined him in his medical research.[93] Physicians recognized that reaching individuals who were not seen in clinics or professional practice was essential to disease prevention, effectively requiring use of print-based mass media at the start of the twentieth century. With the rise in literacy rates in the late nineteenth century, an increasing number of young people would have been able to read the Society's warnings. While it has been conventional to regard literacy as a marker of social class or a norm possible only among an educated elite, it is also possible to see the awareness of young readers in Fournier's personal life.

Fournier's observations on adolescence were formed, at least in part, through conversations with the young people in his family circle. At a celebration of the fiftieth anniversary of the Society, his successor at the hospital quoted the recollections of Fournier's granddaughter, who described the noted physician as a devoted and involved family elder: "He loved young people and knew how to put up with them; he was quite interested in us, his granddaughters. . . . He wanted us to read, asked about our lessons and demanded endlessly if we were in the middle of a book."[94] She described his presence in a house with exotic birds, dogs, and Siamese cats, as well as innumerable family dinners where his work was discussed and his students and prominent researchers were frequent guests. She recalled how, when she was fifteen, her grandfather directed her to read a paper about his research aloud; to the family's wonder, she was reluctant to name the subject of his research, substituting "a discreet 'S'" whenever she arrived at a mention of syphilis in Fournier's work.[95] Her hesitance, despite the influence of her grandfather and his colleagues, is powerful evidence of the cultural norms the Society confronted through its educational efforts.

Her descriptions of Fournier at home have further significance, too. While Fournier has been castigated for his reluctance to educate women about their health, his granddaughter's experiences suggest that he differentiated between a young woman's understanding of human sexuality and a free bodily expression of that knowledge. He has been depicted as a crusader who "came perilously close to fanaticism,"[96] but in these vignettes of family life, he is a cherished grandfather with an intense interest in his young relations' learning and reading. Nor does he seem to have been alone his interest in young people's reading, which was also heard in the Society's debates and in the advice a contemporary surgeon provided to a young female friend of his family.[97] Memories of Fournier's paternal role in the domestic arena, as much as political and professional concerns, suggest further dimensions of the doctor's commitment to communicating with adolescents.

Professionally, Fournier and his peers knew that if disease prevention was to be realized, young men and women needed information about sex in their teens. The proposition of such education, especially for female teens, remained controversial, but the Society justified its actions by invoking cases of actual young people during its debates about propriety.[98] Studies of the incidence of infection suggested that adolescents "had the right to and the need of our advice while they were as yet very young." Young men who enlisted in the armies of Europe already had syphilis at age 19; thus, the Society recommended that male readers be addressed by age 18, if not sooner. When copies of *Pour nos fils* were available during a public meeting, parents with sons as young as 14 were reported to have "snatched them up in the blink of an eye."[99] Young women who would go to work in shops or factories, on the other hand, needed to understand the risks to their reproductive health by the time they turned 16.[100] Accordingly, a preliminary reading copy of *Pour nos filles* indicated the age of its anticipated readership, just as the title for young men did;[101] however, its author sought to quell concerns about his text by deferring to mothers' decisions about its use when it went to press.

The cost of the Society's publications for young people was at issue, too. Although the pamphlets were far less expensive than a hard-bound book, their price and who should bear that expense remained a topic of debate, particularly when the Society began its outreach to young women. It was estimated that given a print run of some 300 copies, a single tract cost 15 centimes.[102] Society members pondered the way physical characteristics of the brochures would affect their message. Congruent with contemporary concerns about what happened when young people read, these physicians expressed interest in the quality of paper and the ease of reading, a matter affected by production decisions like font, leading, and point size, well aware of the relationship between these elements and the cost of publishing.[103] Because a sponsor had underwritten the publication of *Pour nos fils,* that brochure was distributed without considering whether the association or the individual should pay for copies. Burlureaux was among those who saw the need to make titles available without charge to the young working women who were his cause: their meager incomes, he knew, could readily prevent their access to the information they needed. Wage inequities, he argued, should not cause a further barrier to health.[104]

Depictions of love and sex in the wider world were of concern, too. In considering how to inculcate proper notions of sexuality, physicians decried suggestive images used in street-side advertisements for theatrical performances and novels that portrayed romantic feelings in too much detail. Despite these misgivings, the Society nonetheless hoped journalistic and literary communications could be turned to the advantage of the ideals they espoused. Nor did they see the brochures written by Fournier and Burlureaux as, in all cases, sufficient remedies for the temptations of modern life. After some debate, it was agreed that the words of a sensitive parent or housemother, or of an authoritative teacher, might aid readers' comprehension and assent to the principles the Society encouraged, yet it seemed at times that even having an elder adviser might not be enough. In keeping with the late nineteenth-century vogue for visual education, talks with lanterns slides were discussed as another way to enhance young adults' understanding.[105] The talks, though, were intended for male audiences, as addressing females *en masse* would have intruded on mothers' careful, private instruction of their daughters.

Sexual and Reproductive Health Messages for Our Children

The messages that Fournier and his colleagues crafted to advise young people about sexual and reproductive health covered a great deal of terrain; the Society's brochures connected the medical knowledge that Fournier had pioneered, the arts, and popular culture, as well as some acknowledgment of adolescents' sexual feelings and social situations. The brochures provided this assorted and sometimes technical content to warn young readers of the ways syphilis or gonorrhea might

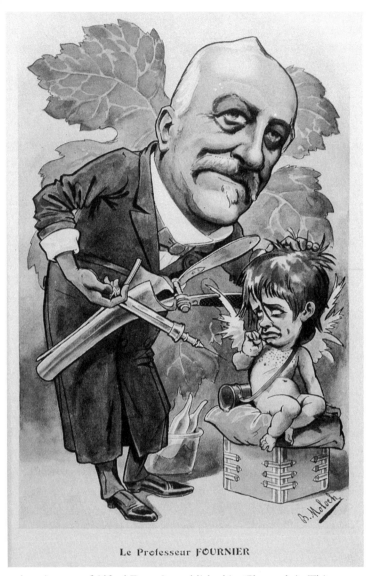

Le Professeur FOURNIER

3. A caricature of Alfred Fournier published in *Chanteclair*. This image and the Veber sketch presented rather different attitudes toward the French physician's campaign against syphilis, while acknowledging his status and his classical education. Wellcome Library, London. Reproduced with permission.

compromise their futures. The goals of preventing incurable infection, of managing perceptions about the appropriateness of discussing sex, and of conveying the real harm sometimes converged in graphic, even frightening, depictions of the consequences of infection.

These treatises described for young women and men alike the symptoms and outcomes of three kinds of sexually transmitted infection, beginning with the "ugly sore" or chancre that Burlureaux dismissed as insignificant, and emphasizing syphilis, which Fournier labeled "the most fearsome of the venereal infections."[106] Its danger, he explained, arose from its infection of the blood, while the absence of this property rendered chancre innocuous; even gonorrhea, he argued, was a mere "shadow" of the threat posed by syphilis.[107] These judgments were supported with discussions of clinical research, including summaries of data from doctors' treatment of syphilitic patients, describing for young readers the personal impact of these conditions. While young men were given extensive lists of the organs and bones afflicted by syphilis and gonorrhea, young women were more often provided with the gist, rather than every detail. The medical or technical material was sometimes supplemented by stories about infected individuals; this young pianist's career was ended, that young woman's reputation was preserved only by an unhappy marriage which yielded no children: both were ruined by a disease contracted through sex outside of marriage. These and other scenarios vividly depicted the consequences of failing to abide by the pamphlets' warnings.

Regardless of the importance they attributed to abstinence, Fournier and Burlureaux both acknowledged the existence of treatments for gonorrhea and syphilis to their young audiences, insisting on the urgency of care by a legitimate medical professional. The case was made by laying out symptoms and long-term effects: the discharges and the pain that signaled infection, and the surgeries that could be needed if disease remained unchecked. Fournier's aim of impressing his readership with the seriousness of the problem mingled dramatic language and medical outcomes. Gonorrhea, he wrote, "can end in death. Yes, death, hear that word. . . . To cite only a single example of this, in eleven cases of acute inflammation of the marrow derived from gonorrhea, we have seen eight of them end in death."[108] Gonorrhea's role in creating the familiar phenomenon of a newly married woman who soon required abdominal surgery and became an invalid was explained to both sexes.

Dispelling the myth of gonorrhea's innocuousness was a significant objective for this health campaign, but outlining the dangers of syphilis, which was believed to have infected 13 to 16 percent of the men in Paris, was its core.[109] Fournier's clinical research on the contagiousness of secondary syphilis would become recognized as opening "a new era in prevention" by definitively establishing its necessity.[110] His later work, in conjunction with his son, linked syphilis and infant mortality, a recurring concern of the period, and hence one discussed in these popular treatises. One of Fournier's colleagues later recalled his conclusion that "infantile polymortality is a primary sign of syphilis, which often ravages the domestic hearth and constitutes a factor in depopulation."[111] A key element of the future Fournier and his Society colleagues envisioned for young people was a family, and syphilis threatened not simply health and career; it all but assured, in the words of these treatises, an empty hearth, a sterile place quite different from Fournier's home.

The presumed desire for children resounded throughout both pamphlets. Whether because of genuine conviction or as a sop to those who criticized his directness on other fronts, Burlureaux depicted the infant as a source of joy for its mother and the center of her life, attributing to every young woman an inevitable longing spurred by her observations of her friends' families: "You admire the affectionate solicitude of these young parents for these frail beings, the development of which is their entire preoccupation; they are ecstatic at the first smile, they dread the first tooth, they watch closely for the first step, and each one of these events animates life and brightens the home. Nothing comforts, after a harsh day of work, like the happy babble of children in good health." He promises his reader that she, too, will one day have a husband and a "pretty family" of her own. Sexually transmitted infection, whether contracted by her or by her future spouse, would destroy these hopes for a family, producing only "irreparable unhappiness."[112] Burlureaux's colleagues pronounced these rather unscientific assertions a solution to the problem of sharing information about venereal disease with young women "expressed in a simple and delicate language."[113]

Syphilis's blight on infant development was described in detail some-times more sentimental than medical, evincing motives associated with eugenics as well as demography. Burlureaux's words to young women lamented the fate of syphilitic infants, who left the family home in a "flow of little coffins." He warned the reader that syphilis would in all likelihood deprive her of children: "Most are not born, poisoned from the moment of their formation, and dead before having seen the sky. There are some who are born to perish. . . . It was better that they were not born. Certain families see . . . miscarriages and deaths accumulate to them of their own volition; a blessing of a certain sort, since the race will not be soiled and these unfortunates won't drag out a sterile existence." Even when a newborn with syphilis survived, he admonished, the baby would not thrive; instead, he wrote, "some will be runts, have rickets, be deformed or chronically ill; may be deranged or not all there, an idiot, or epileptic. In any case, there will be a defect; in some, this defect will be nearly a monstrosity . . . monsters, real monsters, born of you one day, by the act of loose living or even of a single guilty imprudence!"[114] From these harsh words Burlureaux would return to more gentle ones, cajol-ing his readers and encouraging them to resist, for health's sake, their potential roles as passive victims of nefarious seduction.

Despite these vivid threats and vengeful judgments regarding a young woman who had sex outside the confines of a prudent marriage, SFPSM members fiercely debated the wisdom of publishing *Pour nos filles*. Every aspect of the piece for female readers was considered and found troubling by some member of the Society. The membership asked itself whether the newer title should bear the Society's name or if the group could be prosecuted for giving it to a minor without her father's consent. The latter was no abstract equivocation and engendered a dis-cussion of obscenity law, but in the end, no one disputed Henri Hay-em's assertion that the booklet would not revive serious enforcement of statutes against obscene works.[115] The age of the intended audience and the social class to which she belonged, the specifics of disease with which she was to be supplied, the means by which she might obtain the pamphlet, even its title—all these matters were argued, where the companion title had passed, at least as far as the Society's proceedings indicate, quietly and successfully into print.

Fournier had developed the emphatic cautions of *Pour nos fils* at some length for his male readership. Young men were warned that contracting gonorrhea could leave them sterile. The implications were spelled out for them in emotional terms, using metaphors that subsequent writers would make familiar with repetition: "Infertility is not only the incapacity to reproduce; it is also the bitterness of downfall, of humiliation, of indefinite heartbreak; it's also an interdiction of marriage, or if the marriage has already taken place, the eternal solitude of the domestic hearth, the desolation of a deserted nest, of a house without children."[116] A further half-dozen pages explored the ways this childless state would be made manifest. Fournier offered his male readers data from clinical observations that he and other doctors, Pinard among them, had made in order to demonstrate the improbability of a live, healthy child being born to syphilitic parents. Both sexes were reproached with the consequences of extramarital sexual activity; both sexes, then, were responsible for the health of the family that, according to these brochures, they surely wanted.

Interest in healthy children did prompt the sharing of medical advice, as when Burlureaux warned, "gonorrhea . . . exposes women to all sorts of miseries." Young women were informed that infants could be "infected with purulent ophthalmia, if the mid-wife who assists her doesn't take, at the moment of the delivery, all the precautions required to preserve the eyes of the dear newborn."[117] Young men, too, were told that gonorrhea could blind an infant, although Fournier did not explain the existence of a preventative treatment to them.[118] At times, though, Burlureaux's treatise implied that a young woman needed to understand sexually transmitted infection more for the sake of her future children than her own, an attitude congruent with Allan Brandt's argument that such early medical defenses of women's health should not be read as feminist endeavors and Angus McLaren's description of French medicine of this era as misogynist.[119] Burlureaux explained that conventional masculine boasts about having contracted gonorrhea as a demonstration of one's virility was a false sort of bravado and apologetically observed that "it was necessary to make this known to you, only so that you would be able to speak of it later to your sons, to place them on guard toward a peril whose importance they do not know."[120]

Knowledge of new medical findings about the effects of syphilis and other sexually transmitted infections was constructed as necessary to encourage the sexual restraint that had become part of ensuring the health of the next generation of French children.

Dissemination and Impact of the Society's Booklets

It has been observed that the "internationalism" of late Victorian and early Progressive Era hygiene reform warrants a scholarly scrutiny that it has yet to receive.[121] Brandt has acknowledged the international scope of medical research on sexually transmitted infection in this era, and Fournier's research was the cornerstone of both professional study and public educational campaigns.[122] The distribution of the SFPSM pamphlets, which appear to be the earliest treatises advising adolescents to remain abstinent because of the limits of contemporary science rather than on purely moral or even patriotic grounds,[123] constitutes a significant and complex occurrence of "international networking."[124] The dissemination of the titles that Fournier wrote and edited continued, both in France and beyond the nation's borders. Later generations of physicians and public health officials credited him with instigating a fundamental change in the general public's knowledge of sexually transmitted infection that made disease prevention possible. Its necessity and its limits were demonstrated by his 1914 obituary in the *New York Times,* which described his expertise in the treatment of "blood disease," a contemporary euphemism for syphilis.[125] After Fournier's death, a colleague praised his determination "to extract the social consequences from his scientific results" and to make prevention the necessary complement to clinical activity. Plentiful evidence shows the broad effects of his advocacy. His ideas about encouraging adolescents' sexual and reproductive health gained considerable presence as other countries recognized the importance of providing adolescents with such information.

Rather than trying to establish the impact of Fournier's work through conjecture about reductions in imprecisely known infection rates, his colleagues and students considered the spread of his words.

Those who commemorated Fournier and the fiftieth anniversary of the Society that he established offered differing estimates about how widely available these materials for young people had become. Low estimates were that the Society had made at least 120,000 copies of *Pour nos fils* available by 1936.[126] Another account claimed much more. Justin Sicard de Plauzoles, then head of the Society and the Fournier Institute, stated emphatically, "This brochure had been translated into all languages." He argued that, collectively, some 500,000 copies had been distributed. Neither speaker assessed the distribution of the companion title for young women, which was curbed by public sentiment. Even Burlureaux had admitted that his tempered work "raised a veritable outcry, an uprising against it."[127] Despite the reaction against *Pour nos filles,* however, the Society was encouraged by a documentable enthusiasm for its address to young men.

At first, the Society noted nearly every request for its brochures, which forced members to weigh ever-present tensions about offering sexual health instruction to groups rather than to individuals as it evaluated the success or the problems with its approaches. The director of a school, for example, asked that members prepare a talk at which *Pour nos fils* would be given to the audience of young people, whose ages ranged from 16 to 20.[128] Speaking to a group increased the ease and the effectiveness of outreach, while posing risks in terms of decorum and convention. In every case, commentaries on efforts to connect with young people reflected members' convictions that the Society's writings were a superlative defense in the campaign it waged.[129]

Beyond talks to groups, though, it was hoped that a growing network of individuals would speak about infection and morality with younger family and friends. These conversations, which physicians argued could not be had without the aid of the brochures, might be spontaneous, as long as the advocate had one of the Society's titles at hand. In contrast to books, it was argued, "the brochure suits an active means of propaganda; it can be handled easily, without encumbrance; it can be placed in a pocket, because we don't demand a propagandist have with him numerous copies; a single one suffices, on the condition *that it will be replaced without delay by more that will be used.*"[130] The young reader, however, did not necessarily appreciate the travail undertaken on his or her behalf. One member of the Society praised the clarity and comprehensibility of these writings for adolescents, the writers' attention to matters of vocabulary and reading skills, yet acknowledged that readers themselves did not perceive the value of the information they were offered. "Oh!" he sighed. "It is difficult to make a propaganda brochure for young workers!"[131]

Further clues about the domestic uses of the pamphlets are difficult to obtain, but Sicard de Plauzoles's estimate of the international reach of these two titles can be verified (see Appendix A). *Pour nos fils* was reprinted in Germany and Venezuela, and translated into languages including Esperanto and Javanese. In all, at least twelve other countries, predominantly European nations, republished Fournier's texts for young men. Sometimes, as in Ecuador, a prominent institutional press was used. Extant translations of *Pour nos filles* verify its presence in Czechoslovakia and Argentina. Together, these treatises were far-reaching ones with a demonstrable geographical range, albeit with some limitations in places where English was the dominant language.

In the United States, a small private press affiliated with the Illinois Vigilance Association eventually made an abridged version available as the nation prepared to send forces to fight in World War I. The relatively late translation relied rather selectively on the more than fifty pages written by Fournier, amending his text with a conclusion consisting of prayers, Bible verses, and Theodore Roosevelt's statement from an essay called "True Americanism," which proclaimed that "treason, like adultery, ranks as one of the worst of all possible crimes."[132] This rendering of *Pour nos fils,* or "For Our Sons," as it was published in Chicago, owed a great deal to views once expressed by Dr. Valery Havard of the U.S. Army, who contended that in prevention, "the Church and the State should work side by side for mutual good."[133]

A divide between Continental and Anglo-American hygiene movements, long noted by scholars, must be acknowledged.[134] It is clear that the public health campaign Fournier began in order to reach adolescent readers in France was not uniformly or easily adopted in England or America; in particular, the attempt to provide sexual and reproductive health information to teenaged girls was absent from the initial physician-led reform communications in these countries, although eventually brochures like "Happy, Healthy Womanhood" were reproduced across America.[135]

A common contention is that the French were far more liberal in their willingness to discuss sex, but different views about what consti- tuted appropriate guidance to patients caused practitioners outside France to limit their reliance on Fournier as well. Jonathan Hutchinson prefaced one translation with a caution against Fournier's rigidity on the question of marriage, arguing that "the surgeon who, on account of past syphilis, forbids marriage to an otherwise eligible man, must remember that he forbids it, at the same time, to some woman who possibly, if well informed as to her risks, would willingly encounter them."[136] Fournier's dogmatism hindered his cause in some places, just as it advanced his arguments with other listeners. Select Anglophone audiences followed his endeavors to curtail syphilis by educating young people. American doctors attended the 1899 and 1902 conferences that he organized, and professional periodicals provided summary coverage of the key issues they were invited to deliberate. Information about the French interest in educating adolescents about sexually transmitted infection was transmitted via other means, too.

A number of texts, published beginning late in the nineteenth century, demonstrate both interest in and availability of Fournier's research and outreach materials to doctors and reformers whose only language was English. Some French publications by Fournier were available, notably in New York City, where the public reading room of the New York Academy of Medicine enabled those fluent in French to follow the proceedings of the SFPSM. That institution's library also contained presentation copies from Fournier and one of his first books, donated by Mrs. John Jacob Astor on May 6, 1885; the reference room of the venerable New York Public Library, too, held a copy of a later book Fournier wrote for the general public. Thus Fournier's writings were available before Ernest A. Bell, who printed a stand-alone English version of *Pour nos fils,* provided a translation of one of Fournier's addresses at the initial conference, published as an intense red-covered booklet whose title, *The Social Dangers of Syphilis,* was rendered in a heavy, Gothic font redesigned for modern use by William Morris to foreshadow its weighty modern subject matter.[137] This text seems free of the liberties that Bell took with Fournier's brochure for young men, and its translation was aided by Winfield Scott Hall, a physician whose medical textbooks and general audience health treatises later gained significant attention.

Although scholars hail a 1904 translation of Fournier's *Syphilis and Marriage* by New York doctor Prince A. Morrow as the publication that made Fournier's lectures available in English, two other translators had brought out much earlier English editions in the United Kingdom and in the United States. Each proclaimed the novelty of the project and the deficiencies of knowledge it repaired. As C. F. Marshall explained,

> It is a remarkable fact that up to the present time only one of Professor Fournier's works has been translated into the English language, viz., 'Syphilis and Marriage,' which was published in 1881. This is greatly to be regretted, since the series of masterly volumes written by him constitute the classics of modern syphilography. It is no doubt due to the absence of translations that facts which were fully explained by Fournier a quarter of a century or more ago are apparently little known in England except among a few specialists, and are almost entirely ignored in the text-books. Messrs. Rebman are therefore to be congratulated on their enterprise in securing the rights of translation of Fournier's two most recent publications—"The Treatment of Syphilis" and "The Prophylaxis of Syphilis."[138]

In addition to his medical instruction, the encompassing treatise provided an English translation of *Pour nos fils,* here given the title "Doctor's Advice to Young Men of Eighteen." The earlier work to which Marshall referred, brought out by Lingard, became available in London the year after its release in Paris.[139] Prior to this publication and even afterward, the New Sydenham Society identified Fournier as someone whose research articles should be made available to physicians unable follow the French medical literature. His findings were included in their volumes dedicated to conveying Continental medicine to English-speaking practitioners. A thriving print culture was developing in professional reproductive health texts, and Fournier's work was its center. Numerous currents carried his ideas to Englishmen and Americans, even though these remote readers were perceived as disconnected from, and more significantly, reluctant to engage the arguments he presented.

Attitudes toward sexuality and reform movement politics may have been factors limiting the transmission of the Society's texts in English-speaking countries, but its model of physician-led activism nonetheless was emulated in the United States. Observers beyond American borders evinced skepticism about the possibility of publicizing medical information to a citizenry they regarded as puritanical, even as the foundation for such communications was being constructed. Morrow's 1905 founding of the American Society for Sanitary and Moral Prophylaxis was clearly indebted to Fournier's research and teaching, made possible by interactions between the two when the younger physician studied in Europe in 1873 and attended the turn-of-the-century Brussels conferences on sexually transmitted infection (though he was not listed, in conference proceedings, as an official U.S. delegate).[140] Morrow's 1904 translation of Fournier's monograph on syphilis also reflected this connection and the shared objective of eradicating the transmission of sexually transmitted infection within marriage. Despite Morrow's struggle to establish prevention efforts that would share information with young people in the United States, which his colleagues remembered as untiring in their tributes after his death, others promoting Fournier's messages were critical. The introduction to the Ecuadorian version of *For Our Sons* named England and the United States as "nations that do not fear the plagues, that open their doors without any distrust of infesting vapors" and insisted "the hygiene of the country is one of the principal factors of progress."[141] Such remarks signaled the cultural impediments to simple translation and reproduction of European approaches to disease prevention in America; these tides of resistance, however, were not enough to keep French health information from circulating abroad.

Fournier himself had doubts about the sincerity of English interest in his message, despite the presence of a half-dozen delegates from the United Kingdom at the 1899 conference. In response to a clash of objectives, he argued the superiority of his Society's agenda to English activist Josephine Butler's aim of ending prostitution and government regulations intended to protect its male clientele. Fournier scoffed at Butler's "International Abolitionist Federation . . . born in prudish England of

Protestant mysticism" and called on "good French feelings" to oppose its "doctrines."[142] The international movement to educate adolescents about sexually transmitted infection, then, had both limits and conflicts, evident in these contested interpretations of the cultural norms that activists wanted to change. It was not simply that European concepts of gender and sexuality were incompatible, as Brandt has observed, with "notions of motherhood and domesticity in the United States."[143] Other factors, including Fournier's reputation and his discussions with political as well as medical professionals, allowed the promotion of his messages in a society preoccupied by conservative, nationalist sentiments. Advocates who sought to plant his ideas on American shores would not have his advantages.

Even in France, though, the Society's efforts were not accepted without qualms. Crissey and Parish noted that "the French public, especially the dominant bourgeoisie, was not in fact a great deal less conservative in these matters than its English equivalent," which remained in the throes of the notoriously moralistic Victorian era.[144] More than two decades after the SFPSM produced its first readings for adolescents, controversy over sex education continued, provoking the Catholic Church in France to condemn the practice.[145] Messages that sought to dissuade adolescent sexual activity and connected with a more widely accepted concern about declining birth rates nonetheless seemed inflammatory to broad segments of the population. Years would pass before sexually transmitted infections would be named and discussed in the mass media without inciting disapproval, a change Fournier's colleagues attributed to this early campaign.[146]

Still, the Society persisted in its zeal to provide health information and promote child-bearing. It would renew and reframe its efforts to educate young women and mothers, with a Committee for Female Education comprised entirely of women. The committee's emblem depicted Lady Knowledge astride a horse, defeating base Ignorance with her lance to represent its purpose and to suggest the propriety of its woman-to-woman communication. Denise Blanchier, a committee member and physician, wrote a short treatise, "Is It Necessary to Speak to Children? When and How?," and during the 1920s, the committee documented the distribution of tens of thousands of this pamphlet.[147]

This mild and indirect title repeated the arguments of its more openly confrontational predecessors; Mary Louise Roberts recounts its arguments for innocence as compatible with knowledge of reproductive health and its emphasis on healthy infants. Other pamphlets produced by this committee would focus more directly on motherhood.[148] Here and elsewhere, then, the threat of an empty hearth, a metaphor for childlessness, motivated greater public understanding of sexually transmitted infection. Like the Society's original advice manuals for adolescents, whose titles declared them to be "For Our Sons" and "For Our Daughters," these works were equally mindful of the children readers were expected to bear. Yet despite being firmly grounded in values that respected the family, the later titles provoked controversy anew in France, as would translated, transatlantic editions and efforts.

Nonetheless, Fournier's agenda functioned as the catalyst for a network of global conversations that considered the moral and scientific underpinnings of adolescent sexuality and public health. As subsequent discussions ensued, they reflected conditions and motivations that differed, at times sharply, from their French origins. While the forces that prompted Fournier and his colleagues to share new information and ideas about sexual and reproductive health were of broad concern, the implications of these factors were reinterpreted by those who carried his ideas from France to other nations. Their common, often eugenic, interest in adolescents' sexual and reproductive health connected those who responded to Fournier's convictions; their own roles as physicians, reformers, ministers, and writers resulted in an array of publications intended to represent changing ideas about sex to adolescent readers around the world.

Although historical scholarship has linked the emergence of sustained campaigns against sexually transmitted infection to government and military endeavors that anticipated World War I, such efforts began at the turn of the century at the behest of a private organization. Led by a prominent French physician who aspired to provide adolescents with sexual health information, this group was profoundly influential in both its messages and its modes of operation. Understanding adolescence as a developmental stage and adolescents as readers grounded the initial, if cautious, outreach efforts in France and abroad. The leaders of early twentieth-century disease prevention efforts regarded printed texts as an essential means of communicating with young people. Other reformers acceded and brought the ideas first articulated by Fournier and his French Society to their own nations, although they sometimes altered the French source material before they presented it to the public. The result was a remarkable sequence of reprintings, translations, revisions, and re-envisionings of health-oriented material for young readers. Rivalries and professional disagreements also factored into the texts that became available to adolescents and their parents in the wake of Fournier's work in France.

Scholars have drawn attention to the conservative messages found in these texts, suggesting that morality was all and science was all but ignored. Yet amid efforts to alter contemporary values that sanctioned little understood risks, medical knowledge was shared with readers who had access to these French texts for young people or to more faithful translations. Caveats about premarital sex represented only one content stream in titles for younger readers. When considered in the context of contemporary medical knowledge, itself in flux at this time, it is apparent that Fournier and his colleagues revealed much of what they knew to young people, even as they expressed the hope of constraining youthful desire and kindling familial feelings in young men and women instead. Further, although Fournier's tremendous influence guided their inception, the texts could not be said to reflect a monolithic perspective, having emerged from shared drafts and through debates about whether protective social mores could safely be trespassed. Participants' concerns about how to craft these texts reveal the ways social and cultural conditions affected the dissemination of the new titles too. Without denying the strong conservative sentiments dear to many of these advocates, one must likewise acknowledge that some of the discourse that idealized women as nurturing mothers was generated by efforts to mitigate controversy and promote a text with a collective endorsement.

New printing technology had a role in publicizing the implications of recent medical science findings for young adult health, making the distribution of messages more affordable. Despite the costs inherent in publication, print would prove crucial, as the Society's inconspicuous texts could be circulated when censors prohibited controversial discourse in public venues. Booklets reached individuals who could not or would not be seen at a talk or other public events. What physicians and reformers once feared—the secretive text that one might read without others' knowledge—thus became an ally in their new cause. Among the significant discoveries yet to come in this era of attention to health texts as a mode of disease prevention was that these controversial paper products that had been debated, doubted, and even condemned, could make money. This aspect of Fournier's anti-disease messages would be realized on American shores.

APPENDIX TO CHAPTER 1

*International Dissemination of Brochures for
Adolescents Created under the Auspices of the
French Society for Sanitary and Moral Prophylaxis*

BURLUREAUX, CHARLES. *POUR NOS FILLES QUAND LEURS MERES
JUGERONT CES CONSEILS NÉCESSAIRES*

LANGUAGE	LOCATION	DATE
Czech	V Moste	1909
French	Paris, France	1905
Spanish	Argentina	Unknown

FOURNIER, ALFRED. *POUR NOS FILS, QUAND ILS AURONT 18 ANS*

LANGUAGE	LOCATION	DATE
Dutch	Amsterdam, Netherlands	1903
Esperanto	Paris, France	1904
Finnish	Helsinki, Finland	1904
French	Paris, France	1906
German	Stuttgart, Germany	1912
Italian		
Javanese	Weltevreden, Indonesia	1917
Javanese	Batavia (Jakarta), Indonesia	1907
Madurese	Batavia (Jakarta), Indonesia	1919
Spanish	Havana, Cuba	1903
Spanish	Bogota, Colombia	1912
Spanish	Montevideo, Uruguay	1922, 1934
Spanish	Buenos Aires, Argentina	1921
Spanish	Quito, Ecuador	1904
Spanish	Maracaibo, Venezuela	1912
Spanish	Mexico	1911

CHAPTER 2

INITIAL TRANSNATIONAL
INTERSECTIONS

French Texts and American Culture

*He ends by pressing my hand cordially, so now I think that the coast
is entirely clear for us to proceed. I am hoping that you will get out
the book this fall without fail, so as not to leave so tempting a morsel
lying too long in the publishing highway.*

—UPTON SINCLAIR TO HIS PUBLISHER ON

EUGÈNE BRIEUX'S *LES AVARIÉS*

It did not take long for a broader commitment to sexual health education to emerge from Alfred Fournier's public activism. Between the
French doctor's prestige and his work's scientific basis, arguments about
the need to prevent venereal disease gained currency and attracted individuals to the cause. While hundreds promptly joined the association
Fournier founded, others, both in France and abroad, met the recently
declared problem with their own talents. These individuals adapted
information publicized by the French Society in hopes of communicating with audiences who would not be reached by pamphlets distributed individually in Paris. Both immediately and in the years to come,
the men who took Fournier's concerns and made them their own
became, in turn, models for others' efforts. Their parts in the campaign against venereal disease served as the basis for significant subsequent public health communications with adolescents in the United
States.

Although the Purity Movement, a loose coalition of religious and
civic-minded individuals concerned with prostitution and inappropriate youthful expressions of sexuality, had itself gained a considerable
number of American adherents by 1860, its orientation was more to
moral conduct than to disease prevention.[1] Purity Movement publications thus debated sexuality largely with the aim of ensuring its

suppression, and though it sought some of the same ends as the French-based hygiene campaign, its relationship to science and medicine was coincidental rather than central. Doctors nonetheless became members of its regional and national associations, which concerned themselves with the influence of alcohol upon chastity, the dangers of prostitution, and the circulation of prurient printed matter. Purity Movement advocates, in their attention to these matters focused on some of the same questions as other, scientifically motivated writers, and thus cultivated American interest in the questions about sexual health that were first voiced overseas. The interactions between English-speaking reformers and kindred activists on the Continent generated, in time, new sexual health texts for the American reader.

One writer who believed he could effectively place the ravages of disease before the public was the young French playwright Eugène Brieux. His assessment was correct, and like Fournier, he would find that his signature compositions were of interest to audiences in many nations. Brieux's provocative work extended the influence of Fournier's agenda, bringing the cause to new audiences in the guise of an evening's entertainment and a literary manuscript. Brieux, whose writings gave insistent voice to the sorts of social injustice endemic in middle-class French society, saw in syphilis a new problem to be exposed and corrected. Following Fournier, he warned the public about the domestic threat posed by sexually transmitted infections via his play *Les avariés.*

Fournier's influence, evinced in its echo of his long-standing arguments, was clear even when expressed in a new genre. Brieux's advocacy complemented Fournier's campaign but channeled its ideas via narrative modes, fleshing out the anecdotes of ruined lives from the pages of *Pour nos fils* and *Pour nos filles.* In this drama he condemned male promiscuity and female ignorance, rendering medical knowledge of the impact of venereal disease on the family with a personal, emotional element missing from abstract consideration of demographics in professional circles. Written in 1901 in consultation with Fournier to ensure the accuracy of its medical details, *Les avariés* would, much like Fournier's own writings, be translated and circulated abroad, despite generating considerable controversy when it debuted in France. International interest may have had more to do with the play's revelations than its artistic merits, yet Brieux had his champions in that regard, too. Although *Les avariés* has an unmistakably didactic premise that controls the script, Brieux elsewhere exhibited a graceful and restrained prose style. Artistic merits aside, U.S. audiences' response to this French play demonstrates the way documents addressing reproductive health concerns were shared and strategically adapted as they crossed borders and oceans, as well as signaling the emergence of commercial interest in the developing print culture of reproductive health.

At the same time that Brieux put syphilis on stage, American physician Prince A. Morrow continued his professional medical education by attending conferences and meetings organized by Fournier. Perhaps more hesitantly than Brieux, Morrow became another champion of French anti–venereal disease efforts. Following his early professional connection with Fournier and subsequent attendance at international conferences on syphilis in Brussels, Morrow was very much aware of the activities aimed at preventing sexually transmitted diseases abroad, including the proliferation of organizations, some of which—like the one that flourished in Germany—counted their membership in the thousands.[2] This American colleague attracted Fournier's notice, and the New York doctor found himself responsible for translating *Syphilis et mariage,* one of Fournier's most comprehensive accounts of the effects of syphilis on the family, and for starting a venereal disease prevention society in the United States. The tandem efforts of translation and organization shaped American responses to venereal disease, making use of and yet altering the intellectual terrain influenced by prior reform efforts. The resulting texts established both the forms and the tensions inherent in American hygiene reform.

Morrow intended to see prevention-oriented societies established throughout United States; his European colleagues charged him, during the 1902 international meeting on sexually transmitted infection, with starting a domestic association to parallel the ones thriving in their countries.[3] He did not find this work easy, but he persisted, presiding at the first meeting of American Society for Sanitary and Moral Prophylaxis in New York City in 1905. In conjunction with its founding, Morrow described the need for health practitioners to educate the

American public, a message which found adherents in key places. His urgings would be heard, eventually, across this country and abroad as well, as one group, founded in 1910 in New Zealand, attributed their formation to his indefatigable lobbying.[4]

Significantly, Morrow elected to translate Fournier's magnum opus for physicians, rather than his popular works; when the American Society began its work, its members created new pamphlets for young adults, rather than distributing the ones written by Fournier and Burlureaux. In spite of this seemingly censorious approach to sharing health information, Morrow became a heroic figure to his contemporaries interested in reproductive and public health. His persuasive efforts to stem the spread of syphilis and gonorrhea continued until his death, and when he could no longer write, speak, organize, and raise funds to support his imported cause, tributes to his commitment ensued, as did renewed efforts to carry out his aims. Ultimately, Morrow would be credited with the American Society's membership of nearly 2,000 individuals and more distant associations in Canada, England, Asia, and Africa.[5] He, together with a small group of like-minded individuals in the reform community, brought the entwined problems of medicine and morality, as well as philanthropy and money-making, to the United States from France.

Importing Damaged Goods: *Bringing* Les avariés *to America, 1901–1913*

Unlike Henrik Ibsen's *Ghosts,* an earlier play which referred to the consequences of infidelity and sexually transmitted infection—the two were one and the same in this and other contemporary literary pieces—but never named syphilis, *Les avariés* was frank with medical terminology and details intended to make plain the widespread nature of this ailment. Because young women could attend a theatrical performance without question and audiences were almost by definition mixed, Brieux's play ignited controversy. Its violation of cultural norms had as much to do with its insistence that young women learn about the reproductive ills of their potential spouses as its medical content. The dedication of this play to Fournier has been noted, often, as a testimonial to the two men's closeness and to Brieux's debt to the physician. For many years afterward, Fournier's name and Brieux's were paired, mentioned in tandem as courageous individuals who strove to make the general public aware of sexually transmitted infection. Their "collaboration" was widely understood by contemporaries.[6] Brieux, for his part, scrutinized the work of the French Society for Sanitary and Moral Prophylaxis, familiarizing himself with its literature, including its writings for young men and women, which he labeled "admirable."[7] Fournier's colleagues endorsed his support of Brieux, arguing that *Les avariés* was an important source that showed young, unmarried women the danger presented by syphilis.[8]

A speaker at the French Academy of Medicine, years after the script was released as a book, still found the text instructive: "We counsel families to read it. They will see there the consequences of an error committed one day, the internment of a young man's life."[9] This warning, however, was regarded as too controversial for the French stage until 1905, and the government's prohibition was still discussed decades later.[10] Doctors' characteristic conservatism surfaced anew as they professed themselves perplexed by the official censorship in a society where so many parents neglected to guide young people's conduct, particularly that of young women. "We don't understand . . . how one could prohibit a work that shows them the danger," one professed.[11]

Brieux became a noted dramatist whose social reform–oriented plays eventually won him a seat in the French Academy, a credential touted on the title page of published versions of *Les avariés*. Conventionally, it has been believed that little was ever known about Brieux's personal life. His family was "respectable but not highly endowed," and his father earned a living as a carpenter. The family's meager finances meant that Brieux was "only slightly and sporadically educated formally," relying on self-education instead. His first dramatic composition, at twenty-one, was a co-authored play that showed no sign of the social issues that would become his hallmark.[12] This paucity of facts has outlined Brieux's life for those interested in his dramatic work. While it is true that Brieux disdained reporters' interest in his background—he famously told one writer, "I was born . . . in 1858, but of what possible interest can that be?"—he found at least one confidant among his interviewers, who created his own account of the noted playwright.[13]

Brieux attracted any number of adjectives from a man who met with him in cafés to assay the noted dramatist's character: "Genial, communicative, at times rather satirical"; "one of the broadest and least prejudiced of men"; "up-to-date, well-informed, interested"; and cosmopolitan, too.[14] A commonly told story of the beginnings of his career as a playwright involved his submission of unpublished work to André Antoine, director of the revolutionary Théâtre Libre, where it was accepted and subsequently produced. The playwright traveled abroad and wrote prolifically. Brieux's work has been divided into three key phases, from his initial interest in depicting ordinary life among the lower classes, to his concerns with social problems, culminating in eventual pieces containing more traditionally comedic elements.[15] While reticent about his family and his personal background, he seems to have been willing to discuss his interest in social issues and literature with those who shared his values.

Thus, in many respects, Brieux stood in contrast to Fournier, despite their shared aim of easing the pain and sorrow created by an intractable disease. Whereas the latter was an elder statesman who used the advantages that accrued from his extensive education and his social position to argue the importance of health education, the former was forty-three when his most noted work for this cause was published. Portraits of Fournier showed him wearing a well-cut suit or evening dress, the epitome of Parisian elegance, whereas a contemporary noted Brieux's "common blue serge suit" and his resemblance to "an Englishman or an American, playing the role of a Parisian," even when he sat smoking in a café. Brieux never achieved Fournier's polish, nor, by extant accounts, did he seem to care for appearances or adulation. Fournier was a doctor and a professor, Brieux a "self-made titan."[16]

Still, both worked among the people whom they intended to reach with their information and cautions, Fournier in his medical practice and Brieux as a journalist in Rouen or incognito among workers whose stories he wanted to tell on stage. The international attention that was directed to syphilis by Brieux's literary work came about in part because of his passion for the classics, which inspired him to teach himself Latin after he had to leave school at fifteen, a language Fournier acquired through formal study.[17] Their common ground lay, too, in the philosophy that Brieux expressed: "We [dramatists] must have an idea in our plays . . . taken from the life about us, from among the sufferings of our fellow-beings."[18] *Les avariés* was, above all, an icon of the distress of infected individuals around the world.

Les avariés, which became known in English as *Damaged Goods,* related the story of a middle-class bachelor about to marry a sweet, innocent young woman, after he had kept a mistress or two. Georges DuPont, concerned about the appearance of a chancre and other minor signs of ill health in the months before his wedding, consults his doctor, only to be confronted with serious news. The physician tells Georges he has contracted syphilis through his clandestine love affairs and that his marriage must be canceled or delayed some years to keep him from infecting his fiancée. Georges, though, is reluctant to follow this advice; he fears financial ruin and social disdain if he breaks the contracts he has signed and withdraws from his pledge to marry Henriette. He opts for a delay on the pretense of trouble with his lungs and for patent medicine instead of his doctor's lengthy cure. When he and his wife have a child, the infant suffers from an ailment that his wife does not understand. As Georges tries to preserve his wife's ignorance, his child's failing health, and his reputation, the situation unravels. The disgrace and turmoil he tried to avoid engulf him and his family, while his doctor and his father-in-law urge reunion and forgiveness.

En route to this sad conclusion, the play presented numerous medical facts, and it challenged misperceptions about venereal disease. It bore the conventions of the thesis play and its message rather heavily, even a little clumsily at times. A later commentator observed, "If this play were to be presented exclusively before audiences of physicians, much could be cut, and the play be infinitely better. His achievement then must be honored as an act of courage (that goes without saying) and not—in spite of a few stirring and truly dramatic scenes—as a drama."[19] Despite Brieux's willingness to "sacrifice the artist in himself for the good of the race," in the words of the British critic, the play drew outrage on par with *Pour nos filles.*

In France, the production was banned in short order. Henriette was at best a minor character, a plot device facilitating others' dialogue about syphilis and its effects, yet the truths she was asked to confront and the cause of her suffering aroused objections rather than uncomplicated sympathy. Despite official refusal to allow performances to proceed, word about *Les avariés* traveled quickly because a news article, likely generated by Fournier himself, alerted the French public to the controversy. Brieux heard from many who saw their own stories in his characters' lives, receiving "an avalanche of letters," too many for him to even think of replying personally to their grateful, distressed writers. They told of despair and heartbreak, of illness and misery, and Brieux shared their angst. The remedy, he argued, involved opening specialized treatment centers in the evening and on weekends when workers could be seen without compromising their employment and providing free treatment at these clinics. Distributing the Society's brochures that publicized the facts about venereal disease, as he strove to do in his play, was another element of his vision of how personal tragedy might be avoided.[20] Brieux advocated for better information and medical outreach to the working classes, and his play caught the attention of others who used literature to draw attention to social injustice.

He also sought the publication of his play, intent that a quietly circulated text would achieve what prohibited public performances could not. In 1902, Brieux's editor approached Fournier and the French Society for Sanitary and Moral Prophylaxis for their assent to his plans for a popular edition of the play that could be sold "at a very low price." Brieux himself sought and won their endorsement, attending a meeting at which his play and his aims were discussed. Unlike the American authors and producers who became interested in his play, Brieux did not anticipate making money from this work. Instead, he expected that he would have to underwrite its publication with a 500-franc subscription and asked the French Society only for its "moral support." The membership, however, voted to extend its financial resources to the endeavor, because the play "gave syphilis a sort of right of entry into conversations, the same as other hygiene questions."[21]

George Bernard Shaw recognized in *Les avariés* a message that English and American audiences should hear; it has been argued that

Brieux "won his international reputation overnight, as it were, partly as the result of the somewhat extreme praise of Bernard Shaw."[22] Shaw believed "no play ever written was more needed than *Les avariés*" and put its author in the company of Molière and Voltaire.[23] The notoriety surrounding *Les avariés* fostered its enduring reputation, too, and Brieux, who had dedicated his play to Fournier, was remembered twenty years later by the French-Canadian actor and director Loic le Gouriadec, whose *Le mortel baiser: drame en 4 actes* was dedicated to Brieux, "the first master who had the courage to bring to a distressing problem to the stage." Gouriadec confessed himself "only a humble continuator, bearing witness in respectful admiration."[24]

In the short term, Brieux drew attention. By all accounts, the commendations of *Les avariés* encouraged international attention to the play and the problems it represented. A number of editions and translations appeared, inspired by Brieux's informative message, scattered across countries in the Western hemisphere. This French dramatization of national concerns with venereal disease and the well-being of the next generation spoke to similar considerations abroad. It was acclaimed in Germany and received a singular reception in Switzerland according to Shaw, who recounted a report that "when Brieux . . . paid a visit to Switzerland, he was invited by a Swiss minister to read the play from the pulpit; and though the reading actually took place in a secular building, it was at the invitation and under the auspices of the minister."[25]

Les avariés became available in English in a series of editions and genres. Initially, in 1907, a volume of three plays by Brieux, each of which depicted problems plaguing middle-class marriage and motherhood, appeared. *Les avariés* was translated by John Pollock, with an introduction and the remaining translations done by Shaw and his wife, Charlotte Frances Shaw.[26] Thus translated, it made its way to the American stage in 1913, although its existence, educational value, and "universal recognition" had been declared to American physicians in 1906.[27] Slightly earlier, in 1912, an English-language edition of the play, accompanied only by Shaw's commentaries, was published by Brentano's, in advance of the New York premiere, and another edition came out in 1913, containing photographs from and reviews of the

New York production. Each of these American editions has its own story of processes and motivations that led to its production and distribution. Ownership of words and dramatic content, and the relationships between the varying versions of the play, were discussed intensely as different parties expressed interest in making Brieux's ideas available to the American public. Making money, too, was a frequent concern in the transatlantic exchange surrounding *Damaged Goods.*

For all that the parties involved in bringing *Damaged Goods* to the United States recognized its lucrative potential, none was blind to the potential for controversy. Lest Brieux's ideas startle sensitive American audiences, U.S. government officials, prominent ministers, and other authorities comprising "the most distinguished audience ever assembled in America" saw a private performance of the play in Washington in the spring of 1913 before its public debut; their commendations of its seriousness and usefulness in enabling people of all ages to understand its subject were widely reported in the press and thus sanctioned its continued performance.[28]

Stage directions indicated that prior to performances in New York, the theater's manager should appear on stage to counsel the public about the propriety of the play. The manager was charged with telling anyone who did not already know that "the object of this play is a study of the disease of syphilis and its bearing on marriage." Despite its content, the performance "contains no scene to provoke scandal or arouse disgust, nor is there in it any obscene word; and it may be witnessed by everyone, unless we believe that folly and ignorance are necessary conditions of female virtue."[29] The ability to present this argument on the stage, though, depicted for audiences of either sex and any age the "heartbreak" of which Fournier had warned young men in *Pour nos fils.* In a compelling analysis of the play and its 1913 debut in America, Katie N. Johnson traced its positive American reception in order to argue that its performance on these shores "was part of a larger national ideology of purifying the national goods, a strategy that increasingly became allied with eugenics and antiprostitution efforts."[30] More significant than the successful New York production of *Damaged Goods,* however, was the ongoing translation and republication of its text.

By the time a Metropolitan Life Insurance Company official indicated his interest in seeing *Les avariés* move from the stage to "book form" for free distribution "to the Metropolitan's seven million subscribers," others had already published translations of Brieux's script.[31] In 1908, the officers of the fledgling Connecticut Society of Social Hygiene began the project of making the printed play available to U.S. readers. The group's organizer, Thomas Hepburn, recalled being impressed with the translation of *Damaged Goods* brought out under the auspices of George Bernard Shaw and his wife. To him, the new play compared favorably to *Ghosts* in providing "more . . . detail." He sought the Shaws' permission to reprint the play "for educational propaganda purposes."[32] Nonetheless, altruism required money, and *Damaged Goods* would be put on the market in hopes of a profit that would support the developing association's work, as well as readers' improved understanding of venereal disease. After some tense deliberation among the association's leadership, the membership was notified of the purchase of "a complete edition of 10,000 copies to be sold for 25 cents each."[33] Indeed, it has been suggested that the play's publication served to transform the Connecticut Society from a set of directors into a full-fledged, action-oriented group.[34]

The terms of publication were controlled by the publisher.[35] The edition, brought out by Brentano's, a New York City bookstore with a reputation for its distinctive stock obtained from sources around the world and its publishing division, cost the Society more than a thousand dollars.[36] It also required negotiations with the bookstore, which had already secured publication rights from the Shaws, and Brieux, who had to approve textual changes regarding medical facts that Hepburn wished to make. Hepburn both conducted negotiations for rights and managed other, more mundane details of the transaction. Once business with Brentano's was concluded, he recalled, there was still more for him to do: "Several months later four huge boxes, much too large to come through any door, were deposited on the sidewalk in front of my Hartford office. So I opened them up and moved the volumes in, armful by armful, my secretary assisting me. We piled them in my office waiting room with the result that two-thirds of the waiting room was filled with *Damaged Goods*."[37] The title page indicated that Brentano's had printed the play for the Connecticut Society of Social Hygiene, an advertisement designed to promote the newly formed society as well as the problems represented by disease and lack of information about its infectiousness. It was a costly and even unwieldy enterprise at the outset, but one with demonstrably significant outcomes.

The Connecticut Society of Social Hygiene forged an agenda focused on education for disease prevention. Although the annual reports of the Connecticut State Board of Health did not, as of 1908, include sexually transmitted diseases in the statistics compiled for its *Report of the State Board of Health,* in 1910 the Connecticut Society of Social Hygiene formed at least skeletally, to promote venereal disease prevention through information. Its early membership of 630 individuals was larger than some state associations would ever become, and its financial backing by an anonymous female donor gave the group an operations budget of a thousand dollars for each of its first three years, providing it with significant resources to advance its agenda.[38] As Fournier had advocated, the Connecticut reform group focused its attention on educating adolescents. Like Fournier and his French colleagues, too, the fledgling U.S. organization saw the teen years as a pivotal time for convincing the young to shun sex outside procreative, married bounds. During one of the first annual meetings, the association's president declared, "It is, of course, the young, and especially the young man we must reach. He must be gotten at during the formative period of his character and be taught the necessity of restraining a perfectly normal and physiological appetite until circumstances allow the carrying out of its legitimate function."[39]

Free pamphlets, as well as *Damaged Goods,* were intended to make the case to the young, their publication made possible by the anonymous contribution. Some pamphlets addressed a general audience in English and Italian, targeting an immigrant community, while others identified their readers as young men, young women, and those who had already contracted a venereal disease.[40] This catalog deviated from the security of convention. Often though not exclusively, free sexual health texts generated by hygiene societies focused on male readers, believing they must be counseled to restrain their sexual urges; fewer authors were willing to address female teens, and even fewer to communicate with those who were already ill and therefore presumably either in a doctor's care or depraved and thus beyond redemption. As one of five publications issued by the Society by 1912, the John Pollock translation of *Damaged Goods* suited the Connecticut Society's comparatively liberal education program.

It was not long before the New England association realized the success of what some had regarded as a costly and risky venture. Within a year of its publication, nearly the whole of the Brentano's edition had sold, bringing a measure of fame and fortune to the Connecticut reformers. A clearly relieved secretary for the organization reported, "We have more than recovered the $1,100 we put into it. As a direct result of the interest in the Society by the distribution of this play, we have received over one hundred new members. The utilization of this play for educational purposes has been considered favorably by organizations all over the country. There is not a state in the union which has not sent to us for copies of the play."[41] There were other indications of national interest in *Damaged Goods* as well. The Society claimed credit for supplying Richard Bennett, the director who staged the initial New York performance of the play, with copies of the Brentano's printing for the actors as well as other assistance provided by Hepburn.[42] Brentano's publishing rights, though, would be challenged by others' financial stakes in the story Brieux had crafted for Paris theaters. This fundraising effort, then, supported both the Society and the subsequent production of the play, which in turn would be used to promote other printed versions of Brieux's work distributed in the United States.

American novelist Upton Sinclair, known for his reform literature and politics, also adapted Brieux's play for print. His version, which relied on both the English and French titles, was first released in 1913 by the Philadelphia publisher John C. Winston. As the Connecticut Society had learned, money could be made in health reform texts, and Sinclair, who worked to end poverty, sometimes had to contend with his own financial difficulties despite the commercial success of *The Jungle* in 1906. When he became interested in developing Brieux's play as a novel, Sinclair was drafting his highly controversial book *Sylvia,* which also depicted the postmarital ruin of a woman's health. His novelization of *Damaged Goods: The Great Play "Les avariés" of Brieux* was important to him for its potential both to address great wrongs and to ease his own straits.

The effort to obtain rights to work with Brieux's text would involve communication with the Paris playwright and his agent, the Shaws in England, and Bennett in New York, as the parties who stood to benefit from Sinclair's sales negotiated his right to publish work based on preceding versions of *Les avariés*. Given Sinclair's reputation as a bestselling novelist and a reformer whose writings had forced the federal government to pass protective legislation, coupled with Brieux's own status, the potential for profit seemed ever more likely when the story of a young man who married despite his doctor's advice was retold. In the hands of the California author, *Damaged Goods* not only sold, it remained in print until 1948, five years after *Time* magazine had declared penicillin "the new magic bullet" that could vanquish syphilis.[43] Sinclair, then, was a key figure in distributing *Damaged Goods* to American readers.

He wrote for *Physical Culture,* a magazine with health reform interests, and its editor invited him to the opening performance of *Damaged Goods* with the suggestion that he serialize it for the magazine.[44] To achieve this end, however, required Sinclair to navigate the claims of parties in three different countries. Having proceeded with a draft, he hoped that Charlotte Shaw, who believed herself to hold certain English-language publication rights that could trump his interests, would help him gain the other playwright's assent to publish his version: "I will simply put myself in your hands. I have done the work, and I would be sorry to lose it, first because it is a really good piece of propaganda, and second because ever since the Helicon Hall fire I have had to think about money—having been left with nothing but heavy debts and a singed nightrobe."[45] Sinclair tried to convince her husband, another who claimed to retain rights to an English-language version of the play under American law, both of the importance of the project and that it would not decrease the sale of Shaw's edited volume of Brieux's plays. "You will readily understand that if the story is put out in the form of a novel, it will be read by many thousands of people who would not purchase an expensive volume containing three or four plays," Sinclair wrote to the Irish playwright. The Shaws in the end assented to Sinclair's project, as Brieux demonstrated that he in fact had the rights they claimed, but the prominent literary couple declined to make a public endorsement of the forthcoming American work.

Further, Sinclair argued, after the play's success in New York, a new publication would, unlike so many other informational efforts, escape the scrutiny of American postal censors: "This play of Brieux's, having been given under such respectable auspices in New York, it seemed to me that they would hardly dare to attack the novelized version of it in the magazines. So we can get a great deal of information to our readers which otherwise we would not dare to print."[46] Pollock, too, had to be consulted about the extent of his English-language rights, and the original translator seemed content with Sinclair's statement that the novel was developed from Brieux's play, rather than the extant translation.[47]

Brieux's agent, who was handling the dramatist's correspondence, further complicated the tangled issue of international rights, first by unknowingly committing errors in his application for a U.S. copyright so that while the French edition asserted those rights were reserved to the author, they could in fact be claimed by others.[48] Marcel Ballot, in his capacity as literary agent, imposed likely barriers by presenting others' objections to Sinclair's proposal and insisting on a minimum of a thousand dollars, paid in advance, as well as a percentage of the profits.[49] Drawn out during months of transatlantic correspondence, the lengthy negotiations frustrated Sinclair, who worried his publication would be pre-empted by someone else's edition.[50] Brieux eventually took over these negotiations and endorsed the project in a long, "very cordial" letter, written in "very illegible French" in exchange for some compensation.[51] As Sinclair told his publisher, "He ends by pressing my hand cordially, so now I think that the coast is entirely clear for us to proceed. I am hoping that you will get out the book this fall without fail, so as not to leave so tempting a morsel lying too long in the publishing highway."[52] It was becoming common knowledge that Brentano's, having published the edition of *Damaged Goods* for the Connecticut Society for Social Hygiene, was preparing its own forty-cent edition, with the potential to undercut the market for Sinclair's work.[53]

In late 1913, the John C. Winston Company published *Damaged Goods: The Great Play "Les avariés" of Brieux*. The choice of publisher was strategic, linked to the company's back list of Bibles and religious books; Sinclair trusted that the honorable John Winston, "if any one, can persuade the general public to take 'Damaged Goods' as a matter of education rather than sensation."[54] Yet he aspired to realize a marketing sensation, with his publisher's help. In a letter that told Winston that the revised manuscript would be "on the next steamer," the author pleaded for advertising and promotion for *Damaged Goods*. "Everyone I know is of the opinion that the story ought to have a large sale—larger than my books have. The reasons are the play and its success, and the continually spreading interest in the subject," Sinclair asserted.[55]

Bennett knew this, too, and voiced some objections. Although he approved of the project and consented, in exchange for a percentage, to allow photographs of his production to be used, he still complained to Winston, "Your object seems to be not to sell this novel on its merits but on the strength of the advertising that I am giving 'Damaged Goods' throughout the country. Of course, you must take into consideration that to Mrs. Bernard Shaw is due the introduction of 'Damaged Goods' into this country; to Mr. Richard Bennett and Co-Workers is due its popularity." Not content with this pronouncement, Bennett indicated that 3 percent of his profits on the play were being given "to sociology" and suggested that Sinclair do the same.[56] Once done with his lecturing, however, Bennett granted exclusive rights for the use of photos and other documents that testified to the play's merits. He hoped that the combination of Sinclair's name and his publicity would produce a compelling product. Finally, he advised Winston via Western Union, "If you have these books out by November third send me a batch of them to Cincinnati care of Grand Opera House. I think I can sell eight hundred copies in Cincinnati. Then you better get busy on Kansas City."[57]

In print at last, Sinclair promised his American readers and the play's original author alike that his aim was to produce a faithful text, but this claim was belied by a number of subtle and curious changes. "My endeavor has been to tell a simple story, preserving as closely as possible the spirit and feeling of the original," Sinclair stated in a preface to the book.[58] Yet he felt obligated to explain French culture to his American readers, spending pages of the novel on phenomena like the *mariage de convenance*. Even more curiously, Sinclair also provided multiple clues that, just a decade after the publication of the French *Pour nos fils* pamphlets, the reading of sexual health materials was becoming normal and even accepted.

Where Brieux's protagonist consulted a doctor for information, Sinclair's consulted books. Literature tempted George and opened his eyes to a knowledge he soon regretted. The George whom American readers encountered in Sinclair's novel first learned of the "irregular relationships" that reformers regarded as the gateway to infection "in the books he read and plays he saw." In these sources, "George found everything to encourage him to think it was a romantic and delightful thing to keep up a secret intrigue." Having lured him into premarital relationships, books also fed his concerns about the health consequences of his actions. He discusses his fears of infection indirectly with a friend, who replies: "And yet . . . according to the books, it isn't so uncommon." As his marriage approaches, George buys first one medical book about venereal disease, then more, and when his doctor reproaches him for his callowness, he does so by reading his patient a description of the course of the disease from a medical text. The same source will torment George later, when he nervously awaits the birth of his first child: "He remembered all the dreadful monstrosities of which he had read—infants that were born of syphilitic parents."[59] As well as depicting disease's effects on young people, Sinclair's revision documented the development of a print culture that made medical information available to common—and particularly young—readers.

Morrow's Model for American Social Hygiene

Given such energetic efforts to convey *Damaged Goods* to American audiences, the laborious process of forming an American group comparable to the French Society for Sanitary and Moral Prophylaxis, occurring at roughly the same time, can appear odd, even contradictory.

Yet winning physicians and public health officials to the cause of publicizing venereal disease and informing a veritable sea of unknown adolescents about how they should perceive their budding sexuality was far from a straightforward enterprise, as individuals weighed the resources represented by their reputations, their energy, and their finances that would be called upon to shore up an at times unpopular undertaking. Organizations within the United States developed in fits and starts, with one coming together only reluctantly and as the result of great pressure, while another leapt into sudden and surprisingly effective action. Morrow's own Society, founded in New York, was one of the diffident ones, initially drawing barely a dozen cautiously like-minded medical men together for Morrow's initial address. The eventual growth of the national organization, its metamorphosis into a new entity that would gather similarly oriented groups into a single fold, and its spark to others abroad, must have seemed improbably distant to Morrow in 1905.[60]

Although Morrow in many respects resembled Fournier, those characteristics did not afford him all the same advantages that accrued to his French colleague when it came to drawing professional and public attention to a controversial cause. Morrow's colleagues recalled his "gracious manner and courtly dignity" and "the balanced charm of his cultured and deliberate diction."[61] As with Fournier, Morrow's personal characteristics were regarded as an asset to his newfound convictions. Although he had encountered Fournier's ideas before, Morrow committed to public activism only after the Brussels conferences, then becoming, in some characterizations, "a burning zealot." Others, though, recalled a persistent skepticism, even as Morrow worked ceaselessly toward his aims.[62] With the help of a devoted secretary, Morrow managed an ever-increasing volume of correspondence and a potentially overwhelming number of details concerning the organization.[63] He chaired meetings, gave talks, wrote pamphlets, recruited speakers to address the audiences he could not personally meet, and corresponded with potential donors and other supporters until days before his death.

Informally, Morrow would be remembered as "a humorless man of the highest character" who possessed "no sparkle" but was nonetheless widely influential with other key figures in American social hygiene, like Harvard University President Charles W. Eliot and John

D. Rockefeller, Jr. The obstacles inherent in his enterprise, the attitudes and suspicions facing someone who undertook what he and his collaborators did, were revealed by contemporary commentary on his character: "Morrow was so much a pillar of society, a tower of rectitude and respectability that no one for a moment questioned his motives in starting this strange new society. No one suspected him of advertising himself or seeking patients [or] of a salacious interest in sex."[64] His challenge, then, involved assuring others who joined his efforts that they, too, would be perceived in the same light.

None of what Morrow did to publicize disease-prevention information could have been easy for someone who lacked Fournier's ebullience and charisma, his professionally trained son who followed him into medicine and into activism, to say nothing of his unflappable wife-cum-hostess and vaguely madcap household, all of which supported and absorbed the strain of the Frenchman's efforts. Although more isolated and reserved, Morrow persisted, encouraging American communications that he deemed appropriate, quietly squelching those that seemed questionable. He began with the extrapolation of Fournier's research on syphilis for American physicians, a consequential exertion that drew numerous individuals into dialogue about the implications of venereal disease for men, women, and children. His own stance on these matters would evolve as he quested for more and better knowledge, but those who followed him sometimes faltered in their own progress along these lines.

A Kentucky-born doctor who established his medical practice in New York after some years of study in Europe, Morrow translated Fournier's work into English in 1880 before publishing his own 390-page treatise titled *Social Diseases and Marriage* in 1904, which itself owed a considerable debt to Fournier.[65] In these and other publications he transplanted European thinking about sexual health to the United States, emphasizing, as did his French contemporaries, a connection between syphilis and the well-being of individuals, and the effects of disease on a nation's population. What had begun in France in response to falling birthrates became more clearly a racial betterment project on U.S. soil. Although the distinctive aspect of *Social Diseases and Marriage* was its then novel contention that gonorrhea was an equally serious threat to reproductive health, Morrow made protracted arguments about syphilis as a social harm, in which he moved from describing medically understood effects of the disease to constructing it as a source of racial impairment: "The function of marriage is to create life; the action of syphilis is to damage or destroy life. . . . Even when syphilis does not destroy the product of conception it transmits to the offspring a defective organization—the infant comes into the world a blighted being, lacking in development and physical stamina and stamped with inferiority. Syphilis is thus not only a factor of depopulation, but a cause of degeneration of the race."[66]

He viewed the disease's impact as an obstacle to marriage, which was in his eyes not so much a private romance as an externally governed obligation to bring children into being. The implications for women and children, in retrospect, are both shocking and severe. That a child was born was not enough: "The social aim of marriage is not simply the production of children who are to continue the race, but of children born in conditions of vitality and physical health; it is to produce a race well formed and vigorous, not to procreate beings infirm and stamped with physical and mental inferiority, destined to early death or to drag out a miserable experience of invalidism."[67] The likelihood of children's vibrant health as predicted by their parents' freedom from venereal disease, then, was regarded as a precondition to conception in this treatise, authored by a man whose contemporaries respected him as one of the United States' foremost public health authorities. Morrow intended to "indicate the general principles" and to "formulate as definitely as possible rules for [the doctor's] guidance" for dealing with the treatment of sexually transmitted infections in families. These code words prioritized dearly purchased domestic harmony over other, humanistic considerations in a reinterpretation of professional ethics for the twentieth century.

Although doctors' concerns seemed compatible with those of hygiene activists who decried perceptions of an unmarried sexually active woman as fallen while a single man was allowed, in the contemporary phrase, "to sow his wild oats,"—a cultural phenomenon called the double standard—they also created a double standard of their own. If a married woman was diagnosed with syphilis or gonorrhea, she often was denied knowledge of her own body, justified by a professional stance that confidentiality was the right of the husband, the doctor's primary patient and bill-paying client. Men were told what ailed them, while doctors produced platitudes and lies to conceal the nature of a wife's illness or the cause of her child's blindness. Morrow encouraged his colleagues to build on Fournier's concept of "'unmerited' contagion amongst his female patients," and the problem of transmission was discussed in terms of maintaining wifely ignorance of what was presumed to be evidence of a husband's infidelity.[68]

For years, the *Journal of the American Medical Association* recorded similar debates, where for every doctor who favored an end to misinformation, another challenged, "The education of our girls is a different matter. . . . Why tell them of venereal disease or loathsome perversions of sexual desire?"[69] Dr. J. Riddle Goffe admitted, during one meeting of the Society, "The great hesitation that most of us have had in regard to disseminating knowledge upon this subject among women is the great fear of disrupting the marital relation. The medical attendant is most careful not to reveal the source of their pelvic troubles when they arise from infection through their husbands."[70] No contradictions were recorded, and this preference for stifling women's understanding would be evinced in many other prominent American hygiene reformers' work as well. Doctors argued that ending an acknowledged double standard by expecting both women and men to refrain from extramarital sex was necessary to eliminate the one known primarily within the much smaller, exclusively professional, sphere.

Before a couple married, the matter was somewhat different. In these instances, Morrow indicated, a young man infected with syphilis must be warned against marriage, rehearsing the scenario played out in *Les avariés.* He warned against the "dangers introduced by venereal diseases into marriage" and argued that of doctors' competing responsibilities, ensuring the continuance of a healthy family was paramount and patriotic, too: "In safeguarding marriage from the dangers of venereal diseases the physician becomes the protector of the wife and mother and the preserver of future citizens to the state."[71] In these discussions, woman was valued for her potential as a mother, less so as an individual whose health might be protected with respect for her own rights and interests. Providing medical care, not judgments of personal or ethical responsibility, was the doctor's only course in such situations, which, Morrow assured his readers, were decidedly few.

Such cases would be reduced further by educating the young, and here the emphasis was on the young man. The newly established American Society seemed far more hesitant than the French to address American young women's need for knowledge about reproduction, more emphatic in disavowing female interest in sex.[72] In 1904, Morrow presented what was in fact a divisive claim as a consensus by offering a plan for "a general diffusion of knowledge respecting the dangers, individual and social, of venereal diseases, their modes of communication, direct and indirect, as the most efficient means of prophylaxis."[73] Supportive physicians saw education as the only hope for ending the myth of male sexual necessity, which had been used to justify prostitution and was reputed to be a key factor in the spread of sexually transmitted infection. Self-control was the antidote; Dr. E. L. Keyes indicated a young man could learn "that his sexual yearnings are to be restrained like his propensity to overeat."[74] To temper the male sexual appetite, Morrow and his Society colleagues intended to present such guidance to thousands of young men.

"Each succeeding group of males who pass the sixteenth year furnishes its quota of victims," Morrow warned. He estimated that "every year in this country 770,000 males reach the age of early maturity—that is, they approach the danger zone of initial debauch" and that "under existing conditions at least 60 per cent, or over 450,000, of these young men will become infected with venereal disease."[75] The association had figures indicating that more than 10 percent of U.S. children between the ages of fourteen and nineteen had contracted gonorrhea or syphilis.[76] Preventing these statistics from accruing year after year— "the preservation of the youth of this country from ignorant exposure to infection"—was central to the Society's efforts, as it was to groups operating abroad.[77] There was likewise some debate about how this instruction should occur, but members believed that a range of social and cultural conditions required parents to begin conversations about sex and reproduction when children turned eight. Morrow's Society thus helped to develop the early twentieth-century American market in hygiene literature, declaring that the need for information existed and publishing a series of short titles intended to share the right ideas about young people's developing sexuality.

Morrow saw education as a remedy for syphilis, saying disease was spread through "ignorance, from false and erroneous ideas of the dangerous nature and far-reaching consequences of their disease." In his 1904 treatise, he restricted this call for education, though, to men, and the dominant voices in the newly formed Society echoed this conservative approach. Morrow acknowledged the conflict between professional ethics which guaranteed privacy to the patient and concerns about the health of the patient's wife or affianced but, for all his anguished ink, he told physicians the Hippocratic oath "marks out and strictly limits his line of conduct" in a way that required doctors to protect the privacy of the young men who consulted them and to serve "the interest of the general social order."[78] Under the leadership and influence of the American Society for Sanitary and Moral Prophylaxis, young women's sexual and reproductive health education in the United States remained compromised for years.[79]

Eventually Morrow would come to see the merits of women's education, telling a women's club, "The most modest, refined, the most womanly of women, are not offended by plainness of speech. Their feeling is not one of outraged modesty, but of indignation—of resentment, rather—that facts which so closely concern not only their own health, but the health and lives of their children, have always been concealed from them by the medical profession."[80] That conviction, however, was absent from the initial treatises and talks that grounded this first wave of American activism against venereal disease.[81]

Morrow and other doctors recognized that they could not rely on the mass media to distribute information about prevention. Not only did newspapers and magazines carry the dubious words of "the advertising charlatan"; journalists had refused, following a previous conference, to print stories articulating medical concerns about sexually transmitted infection.[82] Thus, Morrow envisioned the national Society "as a center for the diffusion of . . . enlightenment," offering "lectures, conferences, tracts, or circulars."[83] At the same time that advancing knowledge of health and the body was an aim, it was hardly an unfettered one. The

Society's constitution barred members from publishing any such literature without the endorsement of its education committee.[84] A handful of leaflets were approved, many of which targeted young people. Morrow's alliance with an international network of physician reformers was one source for these works.

Two of the Society's titles indicated their reliance on European sources and ideas. One of them, *Eugenics and Racial Poisons,* made the connection between syphilis and eugenics explicit. In its pages, Morrow argued that eugenics was an extension of puericulture, the French medicalization of infant care: "Puericulture has thus far been chiefly directed to the culture of the child after birth. A larger and truer meaning has been given to this science by extending the application of its principles to child culture before birth. The aim of child culture before birth is the production of healthy children; that of child culture after birth is the healthy rearing of children, both the fit and the unfit."[85] Preventing syphilis and gonorrhea, Morrow wrote, meant the number of children disabled by these diseases would decline. Further, he maintained, it was far more effective to bring up children who were not afflicted with severe health problems. This message would take root and thrive in the United States, notably in Indiana. Another pamphlet would also find secondary audiences. While Morrow did not use the text of the French Society for Sanitary and Moral Prophylaxis's educational tracts, the American group circulated a translation of a Swedish pamphlet, *How My Uncle the Doctor Instructed Me in the Matters of Sex.* The booklet's translator noted that this work was only "now presented in English dress," having previously been rendered in nine other languages.[86] Ten thousand copies related an unnamed male adolescent's springtime visit to his uncle's farm, a site offering many opportunities for informal lessons about reproduction, and its premise would be further recirculated later in the Progressive Era as well. Only one association pamphlet was itself translated, as the Society printed but did not actively promote its title *Health and Hygiene for College Students* in Yiddish.[87]

Responses to these publications were mixed. Circulation statistics and anecdotes shared among Society members indicated that many pamphlets were printed and given away. Yet one lecturer hired by the

Society to talk to mothers and children felt that its popular treatises were too cold and scientific to make the right impression on the average reader. While certain that Morrow was "in no danger of making any such mistake or judgment" about "the kind of instruction that should be given to the children," Rose Woodallen Chapman decided to write her own hygiene literature with a warmer, more maternal tone. "I know the mothers here in New York City are very eager for such a book," she confided to one of her correspondents.[88] She hoped to "really instruct" through the book. Beyond content, though, Chapman considered the form her text would take and how it would fare in the hands of its readers. Mothers, she thought, "would buy it for their own use and to loan to their friends." Such borrowing would quickly wear out a flimsy, meager pamphlet of the sort circulated by the American Society for Sanitary and Moral Prophylaxis, like its French progenitor. "If it is to endure such usage it must be more permanently bound than a leaflet. Then it could be kept and handed from one to another for study," she explained to another hygiene advocate.

Even as Chapman contemplated her book's market position relative to works like "The Boy's Problem" put out by the Society, she depended on her connection with Morrow's organization. Her Society affiliation was proclaimed on the title page of her own publication, and a frontispiece portrayed her with her own child, marketing techniques that enhanced her credibility with potential purchasers. "Mine is the first book which has gone out under the name of the author with the endorsement of [Morrow's] organization," Chapman indicated.[89] Like so many other hygiene texts of this era, the Society's work seemed to invite others to join the endeavor of providing the right sort of text to the right reader, aware not just of the potential to improve public health but also of the way that one's personal finances could be enhanced.

As the Society made approved publications available to multiple audiences and refined its scope, Morrow encouraged the formation of related organizations outside the New York area. Using a biblical metaphor to characterize the untapped role of medical knowledge, Morrow called his fellow physicians to public service: "The prophylactic value of education has been applied to the prevention of almost all communicable diseases with a single exception. . . . The special

knowledge possessed by the medical profession in regard to these pre-
eminently social diseases is a sealed book to the public—a light hidden
under a bushel."[90] Despite this invocation of Christian evangelism as a
model for twentieth-century medicine, only "a handful of half-hearted
men" initially heeded Morrow's call.

John N. Hurty, an Indiana public health official, was among the first
whose energetic determination to fight sexually transmitted infection
would equal Morrow's own.[91] The "jeremiad" which Morrow rather
self-consciously undertook would prove to be a natural mode for other
activists' dogmatism.[92] In addition to publishing tracts, Morrow advocated that those "whose position in the community commands respect,
whose opinions carry weight, who can influence popular sentiment,
institute educational reforms and secure needed legislation."[93] The
appeal resonated with Hurty, who would urge his supporters to contact
legislators and other state officials to show how much an anti–venereal
disease campaign was needed and appreciated by a grateful, tax-paying
public, although he abandoned many other formalities instituted on
the East Coast. In other respects, however, this work at the national
level—with its publication-oriented, eugenics-linked agenda—provided
a template for the work undertaken by Hurty in conjunction with the
Indiana Society of Social Hygiene. While Indiana's efforts to control
venereal disease lacked Connecticut's dramatic commitment to the
project, the state's notable public health secretary would prove, in his
own way, no less influential.

CHAPTER 3

SOCIAL HYGIENE VS. THE SEXUAL PLAGUES IN INDIANA AND THE WORLD

Goethe, dying, called for "More light!" Such has been the cry of the ages, but has been persistently fought by trembling fear and foolish prejudice. Freed from the stumbling blocks of ignorance and darkness, humanity will find its way. It is not a morbid but a natural and entirely justifiable curiosity on the part of young men to desire an intelligent knowledge of the mysteries of life.

—FROM *SOCIAL HYGIENE VS. THE SEXUAL PLAGUES*

I ceased publication of "The Cradle" because it had to be carried with private funds—its message was so radical, laying the axe at the root of the tree—and because I felt that in conjunction with this Society I could carry on a wider work. It takes quite a little money for even so small a publication. . . .

—AMERICAN SOCIETY OF SANITARY AND MORAL PROPHYLAXIS LECTURER MABEL IRWIN

Even before the first copy of *Damaged Goods* was sold, American writers and health advocates had begun to instruct adolescents in the new facts of reproductive health. Adult attitudes toward young people's information needs varied, but they concurred in the importance of collective action and authorship, joining a small but growing number of American social hygiene associations. Activist Anna Garlin Spencer later pronounced nineteenth-century moral education societies the progenitor of American venereal disease prevention groups, but most twentieth-century reformers envisioned themselves as innovators distinguished by their interest in health.[1] Her characterization of continuity obscured the international underpinnings of the later effort, as well as the differences in its constituency. Domestic moral education societies such as the American Vigilance Association, whose primary goal was to end prostitution, did not necessarily count physicians among their members, while medical men were central to the founding of organizations that wanted to stop the spread of venereal disease. Physicians expected that approaches used to counter other threats to public health, like the dissemination of informational tracts in cities that feared the spread of tuberculosis, would be used against sexually transmitted infection.[2] Despite later convergences, however, initially the nascent hygiene associations were independent of the existing societies concerned about Americans' sexual conduct.

The New York physician Prince A. Morrow bridged the developments in Paris and those in the United States. By 1910, there were perhaps ten such social hygiene societies scattered across the country. Their locations included cities such as Chicago and St. Louis and distant western states, with outposts in Colorado and Spokane, Washington, where members regretfully observed, "To the average young woman or girl many things pertaining to her sex remain as a closed book."[3] Indiana was another fledgling site, and efforts to reduce the incidence of syphilis there were shaped by the state's secretary for public health, who corresponded with Morrow and others who saw health and race as matters requiring intervention. Eugenics became enmeshed in the public health mission of both the Indiana Society for Social Hygiene and the state's public health agency. The resulting public/private partnership was unique among early twentieth-century associations working to provide information to adolescents, and its signature publication, though hardly commended within Indiana, captured national and international attention.

John N. Hurty, who served as secretary of the Indiana State Board of Health for more than two decades, believed firmly in the power of print to support health. Once he gained office, he instituted a regular newsletter for county health agents, record-keeping practices to account for the health of Indiana's citizens, and a little red guidebook to explain the duties of public health employees. Other titles followed throughout his years of service to the state, including *Social Hygiene vs. the Sexual Plagues,* a venereal disease pamphlet for young men. These communications, Hurty contended, served the cause of disease prevention through advice about sound health practices and documentation of their successful implementation. Good health as he understood it wasn't demonstrated simply by the number of live births or by decreasing communicable disease statistics; improvements in public health meant fiscal savings for the state. Yet it cost money to deliver this message, a dilemma that Hurty, like so many other authors of hygiene treatises in this era, would confront.

Thus, in 1910, readers of the *Monthly Bulletin* of Indiana's State Board of Health were advised that public health constituted the "greatest of all economic questions."[4] The unsigned column, authored by Hurty, was not about tuberculosis, typhoid, water purity, or any of the other issues that were then the typical province of health officials. Instead, Hurty used the concept of public health to direct attention, as Alfred Fournier had, to the ranging, long-term health problems caused by syphilis. Whereas in nineteenth-century France Fournier had seen these phenomena as a blight on families, in early twentieth-century America Hurty focused on their economic impact. Citing state government figures that showed the cost of caring for individuals incapacitated by disease reached $3,747,429.04 the previous year, Hurty calculated that preventing the spread of sexually transmitted infection would reduce these expenditures. He contended that "forty-five per cent. of the insane are so because of alcohol and syphilis" but that the state could be "rid . . . of much trouble and high taxes if we will only be practical."[5] His reasoning followed Fournier but was also influenced by a growing body of American medical literature that regarded treating preventable illness as an expense to be quelled by informing people of how to maintain good health.[6] Equating good health with money saved was a means of redefining his professional domain to include the freshly controversial terrain of sexually transmitted infection. By expressing French values in the local idiom, he advanced new, albeit intrinsically eugenic, public health goals for Indiana.

In this early sally of his state-supported campaign against syphilis, Hurty seemed to have succeeded by striking out boldly: he called a venereal disease by name, identified its effects, and published the first of his repeated calls for its prevention in the interest of producing healthier citizens. The legislature sanctioned these initial remarks in the interest of thrift, although its members would ultimately reject spending state-allocated resources to distribute anti-venereal disease messages, particularly to the adolescents that Hurty, like other leaders in this area, considered a critical audience. But when the state would not cooperate in all the ways Hurty envisioned, he found others who would, and with them formed the Indiana Society for Social Hygiene. These individuals raised funds to subsidize the distribution of pamphlets and the travels of a lecturer for hire. Hurty acknowledged this alliance only selectively to allies and not at all to the legislature divided over whether to support or restrain his involvement with the sensitive matter of sexually transmitted infection.

Hurty's efforts to bring others to accept his views of health were distinctive, although they were neither isolated nor unprecedented. He studied Morrow's founding of a national prevention-oriented organization in New York and the ideas, whether based on French medical studies or urban social work, deliberated there. Members' convictions and research inspired Hurty to make a case for prevention, which he further infused with eugenic overtones. Both he and Morrow were invested in more than the personal purity, or abstinence, favored by many reformers; they extended this concept to include racial purity, conceived as a means of ensuring that the nation would be peopled by healthy, intelligent, and able-bodied individuals. Its elitism did not end there. The hygienic ideals that traveled across this country in the first years of the twentieth century tended to accord responsibility and agency, both good and ill, to men, and nothing but a decorous restraint to their presumably female sexual partners. Despite these limitations, the prevention messages that Hurty crafted with others would not be confined by his midwestern state's borders. Buoyed by attention to the state's eugenics legislation, awareness of this hygiene campaign grew. Hurty's interest in sexual health originated in European ideas, and to Europe and other shores it would return, via a pamphlet called *Social Hygiene vs. the Sexual Plagues.*

Hurty, Heredity, and Health in Indiana

When Hurty, a wiry, bespectacled man whose every action emanated a compulsive certitude, held office, wide-spread ignorance about nearly every aspect of reproduction prevailed. Although he gained the secretaryship in 1896 and retained it until 1922, during much of this period the average person regarded sexually transmitted infection as a concern of metropolitan areas rather than rural settings, to the extent that he or she considered the matter at all. In this climate, Hurty's efforts to study the limited indications that syphilis was a significant threat in Indiana sparked both praise and outcry. Given many Hoosiers' scornful responses to the ideas Hurty acquired from doctors working in European and American cities, his personal background and characteristic traits, like obstinacy, were important in the difficult work of establishing public health programs.

Daniel J. Kevles has noted that "so much was done and said in the name of eugenics," and Hurty's sprawling activism, which was inflected with the politics and the sensibilities of that movement, reflects that characterization.[7] His distribution of information about venereal disease was one dimension of an encompassing agenda, and eugenics informed his introduction of this issue in the Hoosier state. Since then numerous scholars have decried proponents' blindness to the dehumanizing and corrosive effects of eugenics on numerous communities, but when eugenics prevailed as the epitome of progressive reform, few protested. Instead, men like Hurty were acclaimed for their efforts to bring about change in the face of adverse, unenlightened rebuff. The praise of prominent men, as well as this resistance, offers an important context for understanding the work that Hurty asked the Indiana Society for Social Hygiene to undertake. His use of Morrow's national venereal disease platform generated far more than a parallel organization and literature; it also seemed to warrant his intrusion into numerous aspects of individuals' reproductive health choices.

Multiple state laws, said to cover "almost every phase of progressive sanitary science," encoded his varied aims and distinguished him among his professional peers in other states.[8] His work represented a microcosm of Progressive Era reform activity, including the origins of its guiding philosophies in what were essentially Victorian values of thrift, uplift, and righteousness. Hurty's stance can be described in terms laid out by Kevles, who argues, "It bears remembering that eugenics has proved itself historically to have been often a cruel and always a problematic faith, not least because it has elevated abstractions—the 'race,' the 'population,' and more recently, 'the gene pool'—above the rights and needs of individuals and their families."[9] Hurty's assessments of these communities, his responsibility for promoting the sterilization of prisoners and other inmates of state asylums, and the racial and other biases implicit in his outreach efforts received less open scrutiny than the potential costs of the programs he endeavored to implement.

His activities signaled the sort of paradox he seemed to embody: black-and-white photographs of his thin, typically bespectacled face evoke a distant past, at the same time that his intellect forcefully guided the creation of enduring health reforms. Contemporary currents of reform and the broad reach of his study and employment in chemistry, pharmacy, dentistry, and medicine figured equally in Hurty's efforts to change the way Hoosiers lived. His individual background, his upbringing, and his personality were also factors in developing the approach to health that Hurty articulated as Indiana's chief health officer, and this intertwining of his personal and professional life directs attention to the man's personality and relationships, as well as career events.

Hurty's interest in health improvement was both local and global, equally motivated by his sense of responsibility and his blinding righteousness. His reform efforts reached in many directions, with his interest in school children's health sparked by his father's activism and his determination to stem the spread of syphilis generated by an international movement. Even in his leisure activities, like his passionate participation in an Indianapolis reading club, Hurty brought his convictions about healthy behaviors and environments to bear. His strongest attraction was to the simultaneously abstract and empirical notion of health, not humanitarianism. Although his agenda was endorsed by physicians who had lobbied for the creation of this state office, Hurty's nonetheless frequently controversial efforts made headlines across Indiana, and they in turn made him a household name.[10] Publishing *Social Hygiene vs. the Sexual Plagues* continued this pattern of drawing attention to new health ideas only to meet with dramatic contention. This sort of engagement, though, was one Hurty had witnessed most of his life.

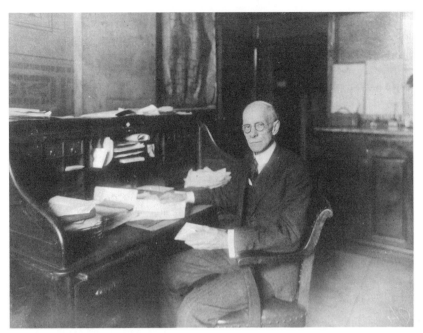

4. John N. Hurty's interest in preventing syphilis through informational treatises was documented by his prolific official correspondence. Indiana State Archives. Reproduced with permission.

The essential facts of Hurty's family life, or his genealogy, have been long established, defining him as a midwesterner and fourth-generation American of German descent. He was born in Lebanon, Ohio, in February 1852, to Josiah and Ann Irene Hurty.[11] His father, a schoolteacher and later a school superintendent, had a rather peripatetic career during Hurty's childhood. Josiah Hurty had firm notions of health involving fresh air and frequent bathing that were unconventional in the post–Civil War years; the standards of cleanliness and health enforced at home during Hurty's upbringing are often cited as the spark for his own convictions. Josiah's defiance of ordinary beliefs was carried into his schoolrooms, too, often to the indignation of local citizens. Hurty once explained what he learned from the dissent that marked his father's career: "My father was ridiculed and received much abuse for advocating and working for the very school system which is now adopted and used in Indiana. He lived to see the system adopted and to know what great good it could do."[12] Regardless of any specific ideas about wellness he gained at home, Hurty seemed to internalize the eventual merits of unpopular professional conduct, adopting the same uncompromising attitude that his father exhibited in his own career.

Hurty's career repeatedly suggested his father's influence, as Hurty frequently acknowledged. In the last months of his life, when he lectured on hygiene at the Indiana Dental College, he envisioned the individual as the product of environment, education, and heredity. He told his students that one's inherited genes and upbringing made the self; these facets of being were the core of individual health.[13] Colleagues near and far saw his life in these terms, too. An Atlanta public health officer who could not attend a 1915 dinner commemorating Hurty's state service shared his vision of an appropriate tribute: "If I were there this evening . . . I would . . . say in the interests of eugenic truth that a good share of the credit for what you have accomplished in your great work belongs to that noble father and mother who started you on your career. And then I have the connection also that you have in that devoted wife of yours[,] one to whom no small credit is due—in shaping your career to its large issues—for good."[14] Thus, the colleagues who formed close relationships with the arch, impatient health commissioner saw his seeming single-mindedness as, in fact, very human. Those who knew Hurty only through the laws and health promotion activities he created, however, seldom shared this sense of the state's health secretary as a loved and loving man, shaped by his family, although this image would have resonated with many Indiana residents. Hurty's perspective on health derived from his construction of his personal identity as much as it rested on public policy, yet he touted the strengths of scientific health management, rather than the lessons learned from his father.

The emergent nature of public health, coupled with his investment in what were then still rather new scientific principles, encouraged Hurty to innovate, and he relied on a broad range of personal contacts and professional connections to construct his vision of a more healthful populace. The loose networks of his era differed from the coordinated structures of the early twenty-first century, in which health decision-making and agenda-setting are supported by numerous national entities that guide policy and collect data to assess the workings of state-level health offices. In their absence, private organizations contributed to the milieu in which Hurty advocated for Indiana health reform: he communicated with numerous activists within the state's borders and beyond them, including John Harvey Kellogg, whose own health tracts and involvement with the Race Betterment Conference evinced values Hurty found sympathetic, and Morrow, whose founding of the American Society for Moral and Sanitary Prophylaxis influenced Hurty's activities as well.

Despite these interactions, Hurty sometimes perceived himself as embattled and unaided, reflecting another dimension of the changed perspective on the state health office, which has since become marked by the need to balance scientific knowledge, media savvy, and political skills, a rare set of attributes threatened by frequent resignations of agency heads.[15] Hurty felt these same vulnerabilities but returned his critics' scorn instead of diplomatically presenting his specialized knowledge to advocates who would help him make his case. The challenges and the strains of this period of novelty and reform seemed to demand the fortitude and other personal qualities that Hurty readily brought to every encounter.

The policies Hurty sought to implement in Indiana were not formulated in isolation, an important consideration given his standing as the "Hoosier health officer." Alexandra Minna Stern has observed that regional eugenics leaders represented a nexus of national organizations like the American Eugenics Society and local conditions, but Hurty diverged somewhat from this model, holding memberships in professional organizations, rather than ones mingling interested amateurs with scientists.[16] He read widely, corresponded prolifically, and attended meetings where he heard noted scientists speak about developments in their research. These interactions fostered his determination to bring about change back home in Indiana. In the state's youngest citizens, in particular, he saw the possibility for creating the better and healthier communities he determined should be the norm. As he plotted these and other interventions, Hurty encountered what John Duffy has described as "the clash between individual liberty and the public welfare."[17]

The norms and values of Indiana, with its "tradition of individual freedom and responsibility, . . . of wariness of government, particularly when it is located at a distance," enhanced the potential for conflict as Hurty attempted to direct the state's citizenry in matters as sensitive as their sexual conduct or as close to the hearth as child-raising.[18] Hurty's entire investment was in controlling conditions that caused ill health, spurning the idea that he could protect rights as well as the public welfare. *Social Hygiene vs. the Sexual Plagues* exemplified his belief that the ideas he acquired from other scientists and reformers should become the norm in Indiana, regardless of resistance from the state's residents or the means by which his aims would be achieved.

At the same time that he worked behind closed doors with private citizens to form the Indiana Society for Social Hygiene, he used the public platform of the state health newsletter, a bully pulpit in miniature, to challenge county health officials to join him in fighting the unchecked spread of venereal disease. The innocent, infected child had been a trope of anti–venereal disease literature for years, but Hurty went further in his quest for a new law requiring, as Morrow had urged, "the prompt reporting of hereditary plagues." Hurty hectored his colleagues around the state in hopes of bringing them to his side, relying on another common metaphor for syphilitic infection, blood poisoning, to condemn the father who passed syphilis to his child. Apparently unaware of the German researcher Paul Ehrlich's experiments with arsenical compounds that made Salvarsan available that same year, he reasoned in his otherwise characteristically challenging way: "If he were to slowly poison the child with a poison bought at the drug store, he would be promptly arrested and punished. What is the difference? Ask the child which poisoning he prefers. He will certainly tell you when he has suffered and salved his sores for a few years, that arsenic poisoning is preferable to blood poisoning. Why does not society class as disgraced, him who bears hereditary poison in his blood, having deliberately put it there?" The dependent condition of children infected by paternal vice, Hurty argued, demanded public intervention, not private shame: "Why does society permit such conditions? We strive to prevent fire, for it destroys property. Why not strive to prevent the fire (disease) that burns up human beings? . . .

Why should we speak of this matter in a whisper?"[19] Like other activists in the contemporary movements for hygiene and purity, although for mixed reasons, Hurty drew attention to the way sexually transmitted disease afflicted the young.

These arguments were the result of Hurty's determined attention to leaders in medicine whose interest in curtailing the spread of syphilis and gonorrhea was becoming known beyond their immediate circles. His efforts to reduce the occurrence of sexually transmitted infection, both within the state's borders and beyond, were influenced by the work of physicians and activists throughout the nation and the rest of the world. Yet the Indiana state legislature, which saw itself as governing a Christian, agricultural populace, was little interested in financing a revolution that would bring information about sex to the general public or encourage its familiarity with words like syphilis, which seldom occurred in print outside the medical literature. Hurty would not be dissuaded by their doubts. He understood the increasing reservations articulated by some clinical researchers about whether someone who had contracted a sexually transmitted infection could ever be cured, noting that this discussion occurred frequently in the context of whether the patient might ever safely marry and procreate. He agreed with the conclusions of his peers elsewhere who believed that the nature of sexually transmitted disease required their intervention, and he would become recognized for his strong-minded hope of seeing that every child in Indiana was born "free from disease, from deformity, and with pure blood."[20] Indiana would become a laboratory for modern work in the dissemination of sexual health information to adolescents and their parents; it would also be recognized as an early and considerable force in American eugenics.[21]

From his perspective, however, Hurty's position as public health secretary presented him with a practical problem. He had knowledge, resulting from medical information gleaned though associations and personal correspondence, of what his contemporaries had come to label an epidemic of sexually transmitted infection. He had data, provided by reports made to him in his capacity as chief health officer for the state, that the rural communities of Indiana suffered from syphilis as much as any major city did. He had a state legislature that authorized his department's annual $5,000 budget, yet would align its conservative votes against funding for liberal social programs, even resorting to calling him a "crank" in attempts to discredit his work.[22]

He also understood how private organizations elsewhere had mounted educational campaigns against sexually transmitted infections. This situation encouraged him to address the problems of public health and legislative strictures by drawing support from outside the system that paid his salary and gave him access to the state's printing press. Beginning in 1907, Hurty worked with other prominent men, and occasionally women, around the state to form the Indiana Society of Social Hygiene, a private organization intended to battle sexually transmitted infection, modeled on Dr. Prince A. Morrow's leadership in the New York City.

The Society's principal product was a circa 1908 pamphlet titled *Social Hygiene vs. the Sexual Plagues*. Part diatribe against promiscuity and part health information, the forty-page treatise bore the imprimatur of the State Board of Health but was authored, and likely even partially financed, by the Indiana Society of Social Hygiene. When Morrow asked the Indiana organization to describe its workings and projects, the dutiful account provided an optimistic, clear assessment of the work undertaken. The Indiana Society had started its work in June 1907. That effort centered on *Social Hygiene vs. the Sexual Plagues,* of which at least 55,000 copies were in print by 1909. As Morrow reported back to the national group, "The first work of the association was to put forth a general education pamphlet. The work of publishing and distributing pamphlets was taken up by the State Board of Health."[23] In other venues, this ready transparency was not in evidence; in fact, the neat picture presented for Morrow's review seems to have been crafted to meet its recipient's expectations of others' perseverance and due success.

Where the aim was not to impress, but to win acceptance by any measure, rough edges were apparent. Hurty's efforts to bring men together to advance the cause of hygiene signaled the distance between Indianapolis and New York City. Hurty advised one potential member:

> The Indiana Society of Social Hygiene is a rather loose organization.
> . . . It consists of about twenty gentlemen who have voluntarily come
> together to do all they can to inform the people of the terrors of the
> social plagues. Membership is open to whoever wishes to join. There
> are no dues. Members contribute anything they feel like contribut-
> ing. We have secured some pretty good contributions from moneyed
> men. At the present time, the only literature we have is the pamphlet
> entitled—"Hygiene vs. the Sexual Plagues" which is put out under the
> auspices of the State Board of Health. We send you several copies of this
> pamphlet in this mail.[24]

Thus, a public/private partnership undertook what Hurty alone could
not. The workings of this Society and its intrinsic connection with
Hurty's state position are detailed in Hurty's official correspondence.
These letters, although sometimes ambiguous or even intentionally
obscure, show how Hurty advanced a campaign against sexually transmitted infection—the titular sexual plagues—that ran counter to the
state legislature's leanings. Further, while he was open about the connections between the Society and his office with established colleagues
and any number of actual or potential allies, he did not publicize this
aspect of the pamphlet's creation to others, particularly when controversy flared. Yet by pairing the authority of his state office with the
agenda of the Society that he helped create, Hurty orchestrated a powerful campaign against sexually transmitted infection, which reflected
both the latest research and enduring prejudices. Despite the state's
reluctance to become a pioneer in preventing venereal disease, word
about *Social Hygiene vs. the Sexual Plagues* spread, and the pamphlet,
intended to overcome ignorance and disease in Indiana, saw national
and international distribution.

When Hurty acted upon the ideas of medical practitioners who
had become convinced that information was the only broadly available prophylaxis against infection, he simultaneously embodied the
state's vision of its citizens as tireless workers for the betterment of
their homes and land, and threatened the Protestant values its elected
officials upheld. Hurty and the Society followed the lead of European
doctors who concluded that the surest means of staving off syphilis and

gonorrhea was to communicate with young people before they became sexually active. Like others identified with the Progressive Era Purity Movement, Hurty believed that prevention literature should warn adolescents against sexually transmitted infection, linking promiscuity and disease to the fate of the individuals housed in state institutions for the blind and the insane. Thus *Social Hygiene vs. the Sexual Plagues* was at once avant-garde and very much a product of its culture, a collective endeavor and a reflection of Hurty's personal convictions, and an under-recognized though vital instance of a campaign to inform adolescents and their parents about sexually transmitted infection at a time that experienced both progressive efforts to change society and individual efforts to resist departures from long-standing social and cultural norms.

It is in this context that the campaign in Indiana against sexually transmitted disease, particularly syphilis, began. Like so many medical men and reformers of that era, Quétel observed that in the first years of the twentieth century, "We find that the general public remained, for the most part, immune to this medical and literary stir. . . . Proper medical information by no means reached the masses."[25] Likewise, not all who have traced the histories of preventive education in sexual and reproductive health acknowledge Indiana as a site of early efforts.[26] When the American Social Hygiene Association in 1940 documented the effectiveness of sex education programs in reducing the incidence of sexually transmitted diseases, Indiana was not among the states whose case studies were provided as exemplars of effective programs.[27] This omission is significant, as Hurty had earlier, in 1915, been recognized for his commitment to public health information by the American Medical Association.[28] Regardless of these historical oversights and the slights of public officials, Hurty was one of a determined number who worked to provide knowledge about reproductive health to young people in the early twentieth century. He did not so much follow Morrow's lead as set out on his own path toward the goals that Morrow and the national society articulated.

Hurty's contact with Morrow is evident, as described in the opening paragraphs of *Social Hygiene vs. the Sexual Plagues,* in the pamphlet's attention to the seriousness of gonorrhea, and in the correspondence between the two men.[29] The model which Morrow encouraged depended on "a local leader, usually a physician, . . . [who] called together a little group of forward-looking people to see what could be done to enlighten the public about venereal diseases and the social and moral attitudes favoring their spread."[30] Hurty sought such men in order to establish a state society whose principal product would be the pamphlet that was eventually titled *Social Hygiene vs. the Sexual Plagues*. In early 1908, the Society had a little more than $100 for carrying out this work.[31]

Hurty actively recruited doctors, educators, and businessmen to join the Society in late 1907, although in 1908 he deferred to "Mr. John M. Maxwell, a printer of this City," as the organizer of the group.[32] Its first members were almost exclusively physicians. At the initial meeting, a constitution was adopted, but officers were not selected.[33] Hurty's earliest correspondence about the Society, written on the days just before and after Christmas of 1907, suggests his reluctance to allow time to pass without shoring up support for this fledgling organization, and the selection of its executives suggested the importance of money for its operations. The Society's first officers were drawn from corporate ranks: John Holiday, Union Trust Company president, became the Society's first president; and Frank Stalnaker, Citizens National Bank president, was its original treasurer.[34] Their importance to the organization had to do with both their social prominence and their profession. Hurty touted their fiscal power to an inquirer from Montana, noting, "We have a bank president for the chairman and another for the treasurer."[35] Contributions, rather than dues, funded this organization, a sign that Hurty expected to align a relatively small number of professionals who might be generous with their resources, in contrast to operations in New York and Paris where larger numbers of individuals regularly gave smaller amounts. The initial efforts to organize this group did not succeed, and in 1908, Hurty confessed to Irving Fisher, a Yale University professor of political economy whose avowed interest in health reform was reflected by his role in the American Eugenics Society,[36] that following a lapse, the Society "has reorganized and started again."[37]

While Hurty continued to recruit doctors to join the Society, he lured other potential members by listing prominent citizens who had joined. Retired judge Lewis C. Walker was among those who allowed his name to be used in this capacity in the years shortly before his death.[38] A contemporary pronounced him "genial in all his associations, a favorite among men, honorable and upright in all the relations of his life."[39] A model of all that was regarded as respectable at the turn of the previous century, Walker and his affiliation with the Indiana society lent the reconstituted organization considerable credibility, an invaluable asset in light of its controversial commentary on sex and disease. Hurty advertised colleagues' decisions to support the organization. When attempting to secure the membership of one apparently reluctant Purdue faculty member, Hurty gave him the names of other professors at his institution who had joined.[40] He also expected these individuals to recruit others to the cause. Edwin Hughes, president of DePauw University, was another supporter whose name could be counted on in Indiana's academic community.[41]

Yet while Hughes was active on behalf of the Society, and therefore a true source of help, Hurty nonetheless seemed intent on those who evinced less enthusiasm for the group's purpose. Earlier he entreated a reluctant Purdue professor to join, telling him, "Why not permit me to put your name down as one of the members? All that is necessary, is to have it read out at a meeting, that the Secretary has enrolled one Stanley Coulter, upon his request. We will meet from time to time, as may be prescribed in the by-laws. You will notice that the Constitution is simply a Constitution and that is all. It is intended to be weak, it can be amended at any time, indeed, the Society can do just as it pleases, without formality."[42] Here Hurty described an environment very different from the regulations he faced in state government and also from the five-point plan that guided Morrow's organization.[43] Without committees and protocols, the Indiana association seemed designed to support Hurty's agenda rather than to provide a forum for discussion and debate, as was the case in Paris and New York. Yet the Society seemed to have retained some vestiges of the proverbial old boys' club.

Women's membership was not routinely encouraged, perhaps because of the Society's philosophy, articulated in *Social Hygiene vs. the Sexual*

Plagues, that women were to be protected from men's unseemly sexual demands, rather than to be themselves protectors of others' sexual health. It is also less likely that women, whose professional lives were almost certainly constrained by gendered assumptions that hampered their equity, possessed the sort of power or social standing that Hurty sought. When Dr. Etta Charles corresponded with him regarding the pamphlet, he did not invite her to join the Society, as he often did the male professionals who wrote to him.[44] Another woman who inquired about the Society, however, was asked to consider becoming a member.[45] While *Social Hygiene vs. the Sexual Plagues* cast human roles in evolutionary terms and deferred to "the Supreme Intelligence" more than to any conventionally Christian deity, its author still saw women as essentially innocent.[46] In this context woman was maternal rather than desiring, chaste rather than impulsive, and most often infected rather than tainted. Seldom, then, was she found on the membership roster of the Indiana Society for Social Hygiene.

Despite the Society's nascent condition and its selective recruitment, word had spread regarding its purpose. Hurty managed the resulting requests for information according to priorities that he did not always make plain. He told one physician who contacted him that it was not yet possible to "give . . . information in regard to the pamphlet you speak of. . . . We are just getting started and nothing has been published as yet."[47] Yet a scant few days later, he closed a letter to a Michigan clergyman who had asked for information on Indiana's sterilization law with the line "We send you in this mail, one of our circulars which will probably interest you. Its intent and purpose is very plain from the subject matter."[48] And in early February 1908, he dated the Society's activities to late 1907, declaring rather grandly, "We commenced the agitation of the prophylaxis of venereal diseases only three months ago."[49] This pattern of denial, deferment, and disclosure when it suited would be repeated in many of Hurty's accounts of the Society's activities. He seemed to gauge his responses against each individual's status, needs, and potential to benefit the Society if supplied with the right information.

One dimension of the Society's work was firm, and that was its interest in addressing young audiences. Hurty saw children and adolescents as malleable and therefore more likely to adopt the health practices and attitudes he advocated, enabling the Society and the state to better realize prevention-related goals. Hurty believed that "the minds of young people are open to receive new things, and are also open to conviction."[50] He described adolescence as a "plastic period of mental development" that was critical for instilling healthy ideals in young people.[51] He told one correspondent, "We think it will be necessary to teach Hygiene in the public schools, and to impress upon the minds of the children, that success in life and happiness depends upon their preserving their health."[52] This emphasis on school-based outreach followed the findings of eugenics fieldwork then taking place around the state, which claimed that "more than fifty-six thousand Hoosiers were mental defectives."[53] Such individuals could not be relied on, Hurty contended, to instruct their children in the tenets of healthy living. Despite his hopes, there is little evidence that Indiana schools were a primary venue for promoting sexual health information. Yet getting *Social Hygiene vs. the Sexual Plagues* into the hands of young people, or to those who hoped to influence the young, was an ongoing part of Hurty's work as secretary of public health. His achievement of these aims would depend on both individuals and a growing network of hygiene reformers.

Circulating Social Hygiene vs. the Sexual Plagues

The paths by which *Social Hygiene vs. the Sexual Plagues* went from concept to government publication to international reading matter are many and varied. No single document accounts for the ranging course of this work, and setbacks and reversals intermingled with success. It is evident that this title went through multiple printings and saw wide dissemination. Its cover envisions recirculation, directing readers to "pass it on to your neighbor when you are through."[54] Significant among the difficulties was the legislature's insistence on limiting Hurty, as he would complain repeatedly, to publishing "ten thousand of each kind" of pamphlet that the public health office wished to distribute. Hurty chafed at these restrictions. "The permission was not granted and no reason given," he fumed to a minister about his efforts to get the legislature to allow him larger print runs.[55] Nonetheless, Hurty and the Society gave away tens of thousands—perhaps as many as 60,000—copies of their controversial circular during a two-year period.

The author of the pamphlet was an anonymous "layman" chosen on "the supposition that it would strike the laity stronger because written by one of them." Yet, Hurty confessed, "Of course we had much to do with prompting the writer."[56] Indeed, the text, which dismissed "lies" and berated "social stupidity," seemed very much to echo the messages Hurty penned for the board of health's *Monthly Bulletin*.[57] The document likewise owed much to Morrow's *Social Diseases and Marriage*, beginning with his estimates of infection rates and his recognition of gonorrhea as a significant health threat. His name was invoked, but not nearly as often as commentary repeating his findings and contentions appeared in its pages. In this often unacknowledged borrowing of another authoritative hygiene text, Hurty and the Society simply adopted a seldom-protested practice prevalent among the interconnected groups of reformers around the nation. When plagiarism and copyright violation served the greater good, it seemed that no one would protest.

The contents of *Social Hygiene vs. the Sexual Plagues* formed an alternately marvelous and contemptible bricolage. Some ideas Hurty and his collaborators shared with young men "between the ages of 12 and 21" represented fairly advanced medical claims. Readers were warned against several myths about sexual health. The author rejected as false, as was becoming the norm among medical practitioners, sexual necessity and gonorrhea's purported innocuousness; more dramatically, however, the harm associated with nocturnal emissions and masturbation was discredited. "The evils of masturbation have been grossly exaggerated. It is wrong to terrify the mind of youth with the formidable insanity specter," readers were told. The origins of this perception were explained away: "The popular impression that the practice is the frequent cause of mental overthrow is based on the observation that many insane people practice the vice."[58] Elsewhere in its pages, the booklet argued for circumcision as a means of limiting one's risk for infection and the critical role of information about sex and sexually transmitted infections for ensuring young people's well-being.

Social Hygiene vs. the Sexual Plagues was not, however, all enlightened thinking. It appealed to "taxpayers" interested in "the cheapest yet best paying investment that can be made by any community," proffering statements that ranged from forcefully quirky to unapologetically racist. Readers were advised that "there is no more reason why the average healthy young woman should be hauled off to a hospital a few weeks after marriage than there is a necessity of a dispensary for cats" and that "man here below is in prison to nature. If the prisoner learns and obeys the prison rules the earth sentence becomes bearable and often enjoyable." There were warnings against marrying one's cousin and pleas to "stop the indiscriminate kissing habit" in order to avoid syphilis.[59] The myth of the black male rapist found its way into these pages, too, though Hurty blamed chemically tainted food and drink rather than any innate trait for the then much supposed criminality. Yet for all this, *Social Hygiene vs. the Sexual Plagues* was a much-sought-after document. Its efforts to eradicate falsehoods about sexual and reproductive health were constructed in ways that proliferated other untruths, but readers seemed not to notice. Demand for the Indiana Society's booklet was constant.

The first edition of *Social Hygiene vs. the Sexual Plagues* was published no later than January 1908, and the final one, at least with funds from Hurty's office, in July 1909.[60] Soon after the first printing Hurty told Elizabeth B. Grannis of the National Purity Federation, "We are carrying on vigorously a propaganda which we term Social Hygiene."[61] His letter established the elements of his campaign. It also linked eugenics and sex education, as Grannis and Yale University's Fisher were among those who wrote to Hurty for information on the state's marriage and sterilization laws and received *Social Hygiene vs. the Sexual Plagues* in return.[62] Hurty offered Grannis one of the preciously horded pamphlets, even as he noted their scarcity.

Interest in *Social Hygiene vs. the Sexual Plagues* was prompted in part by speeches Hurty gave. In 1908, he described reaction to an address he had given in Chicago to another Indiana physician. "The subject matter of my address was sent forth by the associate press, and in consequence, I have received some letters asking for further information," Hurty wrote, adding, "This is exceedingly encouraging."[63] The initial expressions of interest were small, compared to those that began to accumulate. Later Hurty noted the receipt of a letter from New York asking for a copy of *Social Hygiene vs. the Sexual Plagues*. "I have probably twenty letters of the same nature," he observed with satisfaction.

Early on, *Social Hygiene vs. the Sexual Plagues* gained international notice, which Hurty endeavored to support through reprints. His math accounting for the number of copies in circulation was, as ever, fuzzy, but the number of places where the treatise for male adolescents and their parents had become known was tracked with care. In February 1908, Hurty told another member of the State Board of Health that "letters have come from other foreign countries—Germany, New Zealand and Brazil."[64] The list of nations would continue to grow. In 1909, Hurty boasted to MIT Professor W. T. Sedgwick[65] that *Social Hygiene vs. the Sexual Plagues* continued to be something of a world traveler: "We have demands for this circular from Siberia to Australia. It seems to have struck a very popular cord [*sic*]."[66] Another measure of the demand pertained to print runs.

Hurty continually evaluated the relationship between his distribution statistics and public opinion. In early 1909, he claimed to have printed "twenty thousand of these circulars," a figure not far off the one reported to the American Society for Sanitary and Moral Prophylaxis[67] but discordant with legislative limitations.[68] His estimates continually varied, especially when he lambasted the legislature, and at times the media, for constraining his project. He was bitter at the refusal of nearly all of the state's newspapers to publicize it, yet thanked a *Richmond Palladium* reporter for his positive coverage of a speech Hurty had given,[69] and he resented the reluctance of the legislature to fund the effort fully.[70] Although he routinely decried the paucity of copies and attention, it was seldom long before Hurty triumphantly described to others involved in hygiene reform the dissemination of tens of thousands of copies of his pamphlet. The quiet, ongoing distribution of *Social Hygiene vs. the Social Plagues* reflected the networks of reformers and Hurty's influence in these circles. Commonly, copies were given out on some Indiana college campuses and at Society-sponsored lectures, while others were distributed via postal requests.[71] While Hurty's pamphlet was never accorded the spotlight or the funding he wished for it, nor was its chief advocate the pariah he sometimes portrayed himself to be.

Not everyone who received *Social Hygiene vs. the Sexual Plagues* was convinced of its virtues. In 1908, an Indiana resident objected to the mailing of the pamphlet, declaring it a violation of Comstock Laws. Finding himself among the hygiene reformers whose works were scrutinized for indecency, Hurty spluttered against this individual's failure to "distinguish between education and direction in regard to unusual subjects and the use of the mail for the purpose of securing profit from such a source."[72] The challenge turned out to be more of an annoyance than an obstacle. Hurty's application to the U.S. Postmaster was approved, and *Social Hygiene vs. the Sexual Plagues,* which by then had already seen considerable circulation, was officially "admitted to the mails."[73]

Despite the concerns of legislature, press, and the odd citizen, the Board of Health's *Bulletin* reported prolific requests for the pamphlet in 1909: "the average daily applications number 30" and "some days [reach] 100 and over, and one day 182 applications were received."[74] What Hurty seldom reported publicly was that many requests came from out of state, yet his own figures indicate this outward flow of information.[75] In an uncomplaining moment during the fall of 1908, he accounted for the distribution of copies and noted his never-realized ambitions for more: "Twenty-five thousand have been distributed and another ten thousand have been ordered printed. As showing the interest of the people, we will say that almost every mail brings us requests for these circulars. We have sent hundreds of them to other states. These circulars are distributed every year among the students of our Colleges, and we hope to secure enough money from the legislature to present them to all the Highschool [*sic*] students over the state."[76] In 1909, months after denying requests or responding with a small percentage of the requested copies, he graciously sent *Social Hygiene vs. the Sexual Plagues* to a Munich physician, noting that the state had "published 60,000 copies of these circulars and distributed them."[77] A flurry of affirmative responses to requests for copies followed, and a fourth edition was planned to meet demand.[78] These numbers suggest that the Society must have helped to fund print runs of the pamphlet, because if Hurty, as he stated repeatedly, was limited to annual lots of ten thousand by the legislature, there was no way to have accomplished these numbers on government funds.

Despite his account of having tens of thousands of copies, Hurty seemed to deny requests for the pamphlet almost as often as he complied, usually citing a shortage as the reason. To one Nellie Grinsland of Indianapolis he wrote, "I am sorry indeed that we cannot supply you with the fifty copies of our 'Hygiene Circular.' This is because we do not have them. We are permitted only to print ten thousand and the edition is almost exhausted." Hurty supplied her with five copies instead.[79] He repeated this message to writers from Ohio to Oregon, from New Mexico to Louisiana.[80] The blame for this inadequacy belonged without fail to the legislature, Hurty was only too happy to tell supplicants. He provided Indiana residents with the names and contact information for their senators and representatives at the State House, encouraging the citizenry to "urge them in the name of economy and humanity to support all *reasonable* health work."[81] He warned one writer that she found him "regretting that we are at the end of our line in this work because of lack of money."[82] In early 1909, he would tell another requester that "we have not as many as 100 copies of the Social Hygiene Circulars."[83] Some prominent individuals, particularly fellow activists and representatives of health boards in other states, were offered permission to reprint the work in lieu of receiving multiple copies.[84]

Hurty knew he waged a public opinion battle, and he mailed unsolicited copies in a bid for positive media attention, hoping influential periodicals would praise his hygiene campaign. *Good Housekeeping* was among the publications whose editorial offices received what Hurty described as "envelope packages which contain circulars bearing on the prevention and management of certain infectious diseases."[85] The mailing seemed to encourage a favorable reaction from a single state newspaper, and Hurty was grateful for it. His words to Henry Geisler, president of the *Times-Gazette* in Hartford City, Indiana, echoed the complaints that similarly besieged reformers heard from him. "It is rare for us to receive any praise for good work done," Hurty told Geisler. "It is common to receive abuse."[86]

Hurty alternately acknowledged and camouflaged the impending confrontation with the state legislature, even as he sought others' aid during a final attempt to continue publication. Little more than a year after the pamphlet's introduction, opposition had become formidable. To some, Hurty demonstrated bravado, indicating only that "we have met with opposition, and in some instances, most violent opposition, but that does not discourage."[87] Yet to others who could be expected to understand the strains of advancing sexual health information in a conservative culture, he made discreet disclosures about lawmakers' reservations. In January 1909, Hurty admitted to a sympathetic correspondent, "we are in hot water on account of issuing that pamphlet" and asked for a public endorsement: "Would it not be possible for you to write a signed letter to the *Indianapolis News* or the *Indianapolis Star*, commenting on the work of the Indiana State Board of Health in sending forth this pamphlet? If we cannot get a few persons to support us, we cannot continue the pamphlet."[88] He also sought backing from Rose Woodallen Chapman and her mother, Mary Wood-Allen, themselves activists and authors of hygiene treatises for the young, when the daughter wanted 100 copies of the pamphlet—a request Hurty granted only in part, citing the perpetual shortage that would soon become permanent.[89] The truth of his difficulties was also expressed to S. H. Stone of Massachusetts, to whom he confided, "We have been severely criticized for printing this circular. . . . We must defend ourselves before the legislature now in session for having issued this pamphlet, and its issuance will probably result in a curtailment of our appropriation for our work."[90]

Even as the distribution of sexual health information to young men and other activists was coming to an end, the costs and benefits of this work were seldom far from Hurty's consciousness. He advised one potential supporter that testimony to the pamphleteering "work of the Indiana State Board of Health . . . as a *true economy*" would help assure his ability to continue it.[91] His convictions, though steadfast and shared by readers around the world, seem to have been overconfident when it came to continuing to offer *Social Hygiene vs. the Sexual Plagues*. The fourth printing of this publication became its final one under state auspices, leaving Hurty to turn his attention to the health of school children, their eyesight, and the ventilation of their class-rooms.[92]

By publishing *Social Hygiene vs. the Sexual Plagues* in order to carry out a public health agenda developed by national and international leaders, Indiana had become an important, if ethically ambiguous, site of efforts to reduce the spread of sexually transmitted infection among young people. The legacy of determined communication about sexual health was marked by its origins in eugenics, a connection also evident in the national movement's rhetoric. Yet even after the state government withdrew its support for this short treatise, seemingly because it feared his outspoken attitudes toward disease rather than his infringe-ment on human rights, Hurty was recognized for his leadership in creating accessible health information. The work itself, though, car-ried on elsewhere.

At the same time that the state lagged behind its neighbors in indus-trial development and other signs of modernization, Hurty developed a reputation as a leading health officer. While state health offices at the turn of the previous century have been described as "largely powerless and ineffective," Hurty, for good and ill, defied this characterization repeatedly.[93] His fellow health professionals recognized that his relent-less energy and attention to matters of well-being defined the potential for improving public health in the early twentieth century, while the citizens whose lives he sought to protect sometimes saw these aims as intrusive, expensive, or even simply unnecessary. It is perhaps unsurpris-ing, then, that Hurty was threatened with, yet survived, more than one political effort to unseat him after he had embarked on high-profile, controversial efforts to intervene in the private realms of home and intimacy with a campaign of informative talks and brochures. The first such attempt occurred in 1911 shortly after his showdown with the leg-islature over *Social Hygiene vs. the Sexual Plagues,* and another surfaced only a few years later.[94] In the intervening years, Hurty had been elected president of the American Public Health Association, one of many signs of how the larger health community regarded the efforts that jeopar-dized his career in Indiana.[95] In 1915 the balance seemed to tip in favor of his detractors, when a bill was proposed in the Indiana House of Representatives that aimed to remove the Republican Hurty from his position by allowing the Democratic governor to appoint the Board of Health's secretary. The ensuing drama was watched by the entire state.

While he kept his position in 1915, having printed and distributed *Social Hygiene vs. the Sexual Plagues* was among the activities that cost him politically. At the same time that the *New Castle Courier* reported that Hurty "gave his celebrated lectures on 'Eugenics' before over 200 men in the Knights of Pythias hall, Sunday afternoon at the regular men's meeting" and a poet mocked Hurty's critics as a sort of microbe to be eliminated, other papers described a rather different reception.[96] Opposition reigned in the House, and the demise of a bill that provided for increased surveillance of tuberculosis patients, chiefly requiring the reporting of cases and quarantine, was attributed to "hostility to any invasion of personal rights, coupled with antagonism against Dr. Hurty."[97]

Money was routinely inadequate to carry out the varied, yet nearly invariably eugenic, health agendas that he considered necessary for the state's improvement. Printing costs for *Social Hygiene vs. the Sexual Plagues* and other health promotion messages repeatedly exceeded the budget Hurty had for these expenditures. He complained to one writer whom he hoped would petition the legislature in support of his budget increases, "It would be an economy, for it is obvious if the public health can be uplifted even one per cent, that the people will be made more prosperous and happy, for does not all our happiness and wealth depend upon our health?"[98]

Vital statistics were another of his signature interests. He insisted on registering births and deaths in Indiana and spoke on the subject at a national meeting of health officials.[99] The state's *Monthly Bulletin,* under his editorship, regularly published these statistics as well as restatements of the rules and complaints against those who were reluctant to comply. These rearticulations suggest that at least some Hoosiers found complying with this health edict troublesome. Certainly, there is evidence that Hurty's data collection was more comprehensive than that of other states during this time. Beyond raw numbers and insistence on their importance, Hurty also commented on the trends that they represented. To him, the figures measured whether the state's residents were more susceptible to disease than to reason:

Had the messages he created in conjunction with the Indiana Society for Social Hygiene been received? Or did the figures of disease and death that county officials compiled suggest the critical pamphlet had not reached enough readers?

Statistical reports, though, were not enough to occupy Hurty. With *Social Hygiene vs. the Sexual Plagues* banished to obscurity by the legislature's refusal to furnish printing costs, he turned his attention elsewhere. In 1914, he published the *Indiana Mothers' Baby Book,* a treatise on healthful child-raising that informed related outreach efforts such as the Better Babies Contest at the Indiana State Fair.[100] These endeavors in infant hygiene, like many of Hurty's projects, reflected an amalgam of his previously developed philosophies of well-being and national programs. In this instance, Hurty's *Baby Book* brought forward the eugenic orientation of his anti–venereal disease campaigns—the much-noted Child Creed asserting children's "right to be born free of disease" first appeared as a 1910 article he wrote for the Indiana State Board of Health's *Monthly Bulletin.*[101] At the same time that he promoted an agenda developed earlier in his career, he now connected those interests to a larger and better-funded national health program. Although the state-based programs were resisted by a number of associations who opposed the legislation as it was heard in Congress, Hurty was able, by declaring strong support for healthy mothers and babies, to use its funds to establish a division of Infant and Child Hygiene within his purview.[102] The division, in turn, propagated his revised perspective on reproductive health.

He retired from his position with the state only three years before his death; further accolades, though none with the fervor of 1915, followed his resignation. The voices that touted his accomplishments described Hurty as forward-looking, seeing possibilities for well-being where disease had prevailed; yet many were aware that some of his official actions, always contentious, were being scrutinized by the Indiana Supreme Court.

Social Hygiene vs. the Sexual Plagues was not the extent of Hurty's views about reproduction, and the strictures he disseminated to adolescent readers were only one component of an agenda that even some contemporaries found troubling. Around the nation, Hurty became known for curtailing the child-bearing of people regarded as undesirable. Residents of other states and nations consulted him about Indiana's marriage and sterilization laws, which were passed with his support to enforce eugenic limitations on reproduction early in the twentieth century. The first of these laws restricting marriage was passed in 1905, followed by one permitting sterilization of the incarcerated and the institutionalized.[103] Both laws targeted individuals convicted of criminal offenses, whether major or minor, as well as those who were deemed mentally or morally deficient. Many who queried Hurty on this subject received copies of *Social Hygiene vs. the Sexual Plagues* in response to their questions about the state's legislation. The sterilization law lost official sanction shortly after its enactment, when the state's next Democratic governor, Thomas R. Marshall, issued an executive order against institutional sterilization in 1909.[104]

Hurty's 1922 resignation from the state position that he occupied for more than a quarter of a century has been explained with his statement that "it was time for 'a man of another temperament to take over the work.'"[105] His departure preceded, by very few years, his death; like Morrow and some of the other leaders of the early twentieth-century hygiene movement, Hurty used the status and the seniority he had gained throughout a lifetime of work to advocate for aims that were both controversial and beneficial. It must be observed, however, that his decision to leave his long-standing office also followed shortly after the Indiana Supreme Court found that the sterilization legislation he had lobbied for in 1907 violated the Constitution. Hurty concluded his career as the state's health commissioner, then, when one of the first markers of his power and influence was overturned.[106] That his words responded to someone else's judgment, rather than reflecting his own sentiments, might be best indicated by his next move, which was to seek the presumed power that accompanies a seat in the state's legislature. The lengthy list of Progressive Era Indiana laws designed to promote public health, however, is associated with the years Hurty spent as health secretary.

In spite of the conflict that accompanied Hurty's endeavors, other prominent public figures trusted his sense of Indiana and its people, and they respected his ideas about public health. His continued role as a colleague and a respected adviser suggests that his skepticism toward those whose lives he shaped was shared, rather than being as peculiar as his alternately impatient and insensitive denunciations of any number of individuals might have suggested. Hurty's myriad approaches to public health would see him numbered among "the ten greatest living Indianans" in 1922.[107] Later he would be cited as a leader for pure food and drug legislation,[108] an advocate for oral hygiene and professor of dentistry,[109] and even an "ardent Darwinist . . . interested in the eugenics movement."[110] Yet his equally ardent—and global—campaign to prevent individuals from contracting venereal disease has been little studied.[111]

Hurty's contemporaries neither remembered nor apologized for his adamant and elitist battle against sexually transmitted infection when this former secretary for public health and one-time state legislator died in 1928. He was credited simply with a passion for public well-being; as one biographer aptly stated, "Health to him was a religion,"[112] rephrasing one of Hurty's aphorisms which held that "the Gospel of Health is second only to the Gospel of Jesus Christ."[113] Those who acknowledged his "fight . . . against disease and dirt" were indirect at best in noting his concern with syphilis and related ills.[114]

Competing perspectives about whether Hurty's acts and the philosophies he expressed in outlets like *Social Hygiene vs. the Sexual Plagues* were heroic or intrusive, coupled with the darker consequences of his agenda, suggest the reasons Indiana never memorialized her once favored son. In 2007, one hundred years after the passage of one of the many pieces of legislation attributed to Hurty, the state acknowledged those affected by his eugenic reforms.[115] A state historical marker outside the Indiana Capitol remembers an estimated 2,500 individuals sterilized through the enactment of policies that Hurty advocated as health secretary. It stands as evidence of the dramatic shift in the estimation of Hurty's career, an indicator of why a once notable booklet like *Social Hygiene vs. the Sexual Plagues* faded into an obscurity that removed it from the larger national and international contexts in which it functioned.

Some scholarly discussions of eugenics have attempted to differentiate between positive and negative eugenics, dividing the forerunners of contemporary health promotion activities from punitive and dehuman-izing programs inflicted upon disabled and vulnerable populations.[116] Examination of Hurty's life and work, and the way an informational project like *Social Hygiene vs. the Sexual Plagues* related to a sterilization agenda suggests such a neat demarcation is not necessarily possible. Hurty's efforts, although very much entwined with the problematic idealism represented by eugenics, were nonetheless notable on numer-ous fronts. First, most concerns about the spread of sexually transmit-ted infection were generated in urban conditions. Fournier worked in Paris, and Morrow spent his medical career in New York City. Hurty, then, was somewhat unusual in believing his still largely rural state ought to be concerned with syphilis, especially at a time when country life was associated with health. It is possible that he saw evidence of a demographic shift that would be confirmed by the 1910 census, indi-cating that though Indiana's past may have been agricultural, its future would be urban. Young people, the audience for Hurty's pamphlet, led this change: "Young people voted with their feet and their satchels; thousands of them left the family farm for jobs and homes in towns and cities."[117]

Following the lead of Fournier, via Morrow's writings, Hurty directed his prevention campaigns toward adolescents. His organiza-tion of the Indiana Society of Social Hygiene took place only a couple of years after the founding of the national society in New York, one of the first such state groups. Communication about sexuality with young, unmarried individuals was increasing but not fully sanctioned when Hurty and the Indiana Society of Social Hygiene began their work, as the state legislature's emphatic response demonstrated. Despite local resistance and his own weaknesses, this campaign for adolescent sexual and reproductive health crossed numerous borders. Hurty, who trav-eled to many health-related conferences in order to bring the most recent medical research back to Indiana, once marveled at hearing the bacteriologist Robert Koch deliver a plenary speech. Through *Social Hygiene vs. the Sexual Plagues,* his own words found an international audience and formed a part in the developing, if conflicted, dialogue with adolescents about their sexual health.

Whereas Hurty participated in a transnational network of reformers with shared motivations for providing health messages to young people who lacked information about their developing bodies and feelings, numerous nonaffiliated writers would rush to fill this void with their own books and pamphlets addressed to young people and their parents. Their emulation of physicians' health writings for adolescents prompted new responses to such texts that belied publishers' ability to capitalize on the establishing market for sexual and reproductive health titles. Their for-profit works displayed their eugenics themes more lightly, while insisting more fervently that they gave voice to God's pronouncements on creation and procreation. Resolving reformers' dilemmas related to the costs of producing texts for young people left a new contingent of writers to confront other problems that were perhaps inherent in providing information on reproduction to Progressive Era adolescents.

CHAPTER 4

WHAT YOUNG READERS OUGHT TO KNOW

The Successful Selling of Sex Education

Like the railroad tracks that have carried the engines and trains of modern thought, civilization, and progress, these more than 5,000 miles of priceless information have regenerated and saved thousands upon thousands who were groping blindly in disease and ignorance.

—L. M. CROSS ON THE SELF AND SEX SERIES

Neither the difficulties of financing sexual health education nor its progressive mission could forestall reproaches against the growing body of informative treatises. "There is nothing new about the Seven Deadly Sins," Agnes Repellier wrote in 1916. Her apologia for innocence and decency, "The Repeal of Reticence," recoiled from the attention that the Purity Movement and related reform efforts gave to sex and the body. Repellier, a prominent writer for the *Atlantic Monthly,* found the resulting public discourse distasteful: "Why then do so many men and women talk and write as if they had just discovered these ancient associates of mankind? Why do they press upon our reluctant notice the result of their researches? Why this fresh enthusiasm for a foul subject? Why this relentless determination to make us intimately acquainted with matters of which a casual knowledge would suffice?" Among those whom she singled out for contempt were the "self-appointed instructors" and "ardent but uninstructed missionaries." Labeling the discussion of hygiene missionary work was, to her, mere dissembling, and claiming that young people were naturally curious about sex and the body was a falsehood. Repellier believed that even "those who first cautiously advised a clearer understanding of sexual relations and hygienic laws" did not intend their advocacy to result in strangers on one's doorstep offering such information. "What can be thought of a woman who goes to a household of strangers, and volunteers to instruct its members in sex-hygiene!" she demanded.[1] Her own response to such an outrage was clear.

Her ardent complaint against the traveling hygiene missionary would surely have troubled the Reverend Sylvanus Stall, had he been alive to read her words. Stall, who died in 1915, was ordained as a Lutheran minister in 1874 before devoting his life to publishing. His best-known titles were an internationally famed series of sex education texts sold door-to-door for years before they were stocked in stores.[2] The eight books comprising the Self and Sex Series were printed continuously from 1897 until 1936. While couched in the context of Stall's religious beliefs, the books also reflected recent developments in medicine and science, a pairing which made them a distinctive commercial product. Regardless of the rather bold nature of his editorial project, Stall regarded himself as a godly man who had answered "a divine call to the ministry" and habitually got down on his knees to pray before a meal, even if he were in a "rather cheap" restaurant where the floor was covered in sawdust and debris carried in on workers' feet.[3] His prominence in the developing market for hygiene literature owed much to his ability to meld religious convictions with an understanding of science and of commerce, the latter developed, he claimed in an autobiographical essay, by earning his living as a Lord & Taylor's salesman before attending divinity school. Stall had also relied on an income from canvassing books to support his vocational education, enabling him to characterize "his entire life" as a "preparation for this great . . . work," that is, publishing titles like *What a Young Man Ought to Know.*[4]

While Fournier and his fellow physicians wrestled with the problem of how to share information about venereal disease without creating a stir, Stall developed a distinctive line of books that addressed the same concerns. With his strategic marketing, Stall proved people would pay for the information that newly founded hygiene societies hoped to distribute for free, though some doctors were discomfited by his entrepreneurial approach to their purview. Stall accomplished this, in part, by linking his venture as author, editor, and independent publisher to two professional communities: the international missionary movement and the larger world of book publishing and sales. During an era when Anthony Comstock, in conjunction with the New York Society for the Suppression of Vice, scrutinized print materials for any hint of indecency, Stall's books explained the relative roles of God and man in reproduction in order to argue that health was protected by both observation of divine principles and information. Cross-promotions, testimonials, sales manuals, and industry newsletters highlighted the reach of Vir Publishing's products and assured potential purchasers of the respectability of the books' sensitive health content. Stall's small press products thus won a place in the burgeoning Progressive Era print market. An American citizen, he created a wide readership by distributing his works via a transnational missionary community and cultivating relationships with English-language bookstores around the globe. Many would follow his endeavors, whether as readers, detractors, or competitors, but none managed to acquire the lasting cachet and name recognition of books in the Self and Sex Series. Their cultural resonance testifies to the rather astonishing impact of his promotional endeavors, a phenomenon whose workings ensured that his curious yet informed perspective would be shared with readers far beyond American borders.

The series' appeal resulted from the messages he and his associates crafted and the way he sold their words to a worldwide readership; its success is evinced by its endurance in the market and the rivals who tried to win a share of the readership Stall created. In addition to Stall himself, other personalities played key roles in his publishing empire. Among them were individuals like Dr. Mary Wood-Allen, who contributed to the series' success through her authorship and her alignment with coalitions including the Woman's Christian Temperance Union and the National Purity Federation, and Dr. Winfield Scott Hall, who sought to supplant Stall's position as the market leader. Because both Wood-Allen and Hall were prominent figures in contemporary hygiene reform who had articulated their views on sex, race, and nationalism as factors in individual health before national audiences, they drew attention in their own right, rather than simply through their relationship to Stall. Stall's hygiene titles, however, delivered their ideas to a new readership of adolescents and their parents, undergirded by his own strong commercial motives. Publication of the Self and Sex Series continued even after Stall no longer controlled its tone and advertising, as did its competition, another indication of the popular appeal of rather conservative hygiene treatises that emphasized traditional values rather than the frank presentation of medical facts.

Stall's Series, Its Authorship and Reception

Stall's road to success as an independent publisher was a long, even indirect, one. He first ventured into print under the auspices of the I. K. Funk, and then the Funk and Wagnalls, companies with titles for ministers. These initial books, printed in the late nineteenth century but later republished, included ones on the economic aspects of religious activity, *How to Pay Church Debts and How to Keep Churches out of Debt* among them.[5] He was also known as the editor of *The Lutheran Year Book* and *The Lutheran Observer,* and these professional responsibilities augmented his understanding of publishing and of international missionary outreach through travel abroad.[6] As Funk and Wagnalls developed a more secular orientation, Stall created Vir Publishing to produce his own religious titles, including *Bible Selections for Daily Devotion.*[7] Vir Publishing's first Philadelphia offices were in the stately stone Romanesque Hale Building constructed for Keystone National Bank in 1887; in 1916, the publishing offices would move to the New Ledger Building, "the latest modern expression in luxury, beauty, and convenience," near the city's publishing center and Independence Square.[8] From this domestic location in a city long known for medical publishing, Vir Publishing became a tri-national company with facilities in London and in Toronto, where it was affiliated with the William Briggs Company, which also published the commercially successful wilderness poetry of Robert Service—author of "The Shooting of Dan McGrew"—during these years. Simultaneously with this international move, Stall had begun the work for which he would ultimately be remembered.

The Self and Sex Series, whose titles proclaimed a commonsense authority that became emblematic of self-read sex education, comprised Vir Publishing's principal hygiene works, although other treatises were added to the company's roster. To the public, Stall characterized these books as the result of a vow he had made to God and himself to address the anxious feelings of youth. His approach was a compelling one. A review of *What a Young Man Ought to Know* apprised potential readers that Stall's "pure and invaluable series" addressed "delicate but important questions . . . in a plain, practical, and most satisfactory manner." The reviewer marveled that the result was books that "differ from anything else ever attempted in English.[9] Among the turn-of-the-century efforts to turn the parent-child conversation about the facts of life into a print industry, Stall's workings were indeed distinctive. In contrast to the dark, elaborate Victorian covers of sensationally moralistic tomes and the thin pamphlets commonly produced by private organizations founded solely to fight venereal disease, Stall brought a minister's point of view—and, significantly, his credentials—to the discussion of modern medical facts. Books in the Self and Sex Series typically offered health information that would have been accepted by contemporary physicians, but their authors also demonstrated the importance of living in accord with conventional religious values. Such a life centered on a marriage that would produce healthy, happy Christian babies. Despite the consistency with which Stall articulated this perspective, one radical contemporary vacillated in his opinion of Stall's work, sometimes differentiating the Self and Sex Series from the mass of books which he criticized as "Christian fictions about sex" and at others seeming to praise Stall as the "author and publisher of numerous sexy books on what people of all ages ought to know."[10] Whether because of its brand of discreet sexiness or its conservatism, this guidance, produced during Stall's lifetime as red hardcover books with gold-embossed lettering, sold.

At a dollar per book, the going rate for any new general audience book of this era, works in the Self and Sex Series contained elements designed to convey their necessity and decency to potential purchasers.[11] At the same time, however, the books cost at least a dollar less than other success manuals sold door-to-door.[12] Over time, the books' price would rise, but the base price of a dollar remained a selling point, as when thirtieth-anniversary editions retailed for their introductory price once more.[13] Stall's production decisions were designed to allay common concerns about the immoral content of cheap literature. Further, Stall contended that this form could be sold via newsstands and booksellers, whereas pamphlet literature could not.[14] The books' format, then, was intended to enhance marketability in multiple ways. His works shared the form of respectable, or at least uncontroversial books, but readers were not left to judge the books in the series by their covers.

The books began with photographs and testimonials from "Eminent Men and Women."[15] This strategy, used to sell other contemporary conduct manuals, would become important as a protective convention in American social hygiene literature.[16] One edition of *What a Young Man Ought to Know* was recommended by no fewer than eighteen individuals before readers even encountered a title page.[17] Most who provided testimonials were doctors and ministers, but W. H. P. Faunce, president of Brown University, and John W. Philip, admiral of the U.S. Navy, also supplied their praise. Stall would make much of the naval endorsement and the inclusion of *What a Young Man Ought to Know* in ships' libraries. The texts for women were endorsed by suffragist Elizabeth Cady Stanton, who saw these books as staving off social and moral ruin: "The life of many a boy and girl is totally wrecked through the abuse of relations most sacred in their highest uses. As thought precedes action, it is important to keep the mind occupied on the most exalted views of all questions."[18] Individuals including Charles N. Crittenton, founder of the National Florence Crittenton Mission that housed prostitutes and unwed mothers, and Helen Campbell, dean of the Kansas State Agricultural College Department of Household Economics, concurred. "They deserve all the success already their own," Campbell wrote of the series.[19]

Shortly after the turn of the century, Stall claimed to have sold more than a million volumes in the United States and England, with a number of missionary societies disseminating additional copies abroad at their own expense.[20] Stall and his staff promoted the reach of the series as a sign of its worth. In 1915, Stall compared sales of the Self and Sex Series to the record-breaking attendance of more than 68,000 people at the 1914 Harvard-Yale game; he boasted that "it would take 34 of these bowls to hold the number of people who have purchased Stall's

Books—two and a quarter million of them. It would take over 147 of these bowls to hold the ten million readers of these books in the English language alone."[21] Other spatial metaphors illustrated the series' popularity, as the height of the Himalayas was significantly less than the span of these books laid end to end, "which would stretch toward the blue 220 miles—three times the total height of the world's greatest mountains."[22] Later, a Vir editor claimed that just as the books reached readers around the globe, a continuous role of the paper required to print them would cross miles of the earth's circumference. Notions of empire were implicit in his characterization of the terrain affected by Stall's hygiene titles:

> If one end of [the roll] were placed in the Arctic Ocean on the North, it would stretch down through the great Dominion of Canada—larger in square miles than our own country—clean through the United States, though Mexico, it would overleap the Panama Canal, and embrace a couple thousand miles of South America. . . . Like the railroad tracks that have carried the engines and trains of modern thought, civilization, and progress, these more than 5,000 miles of priceless information have regenerated and saved thousands upon thousands who were groping blindly in disease and ignorance.[23]

The internally generated publicity for these books seems similarly exhaustive, but its conclusions—that numerous readers favored the sort of health messages Stall published—went unchallenged.

One likely reason for the books' enduring appeal was their reassuring response to cultural change. Much like authors of myriad other conduct manuals of this period, Stall argued that new problems should be met with traditional values.[24] Toward the end of the nineteenth century, physicians presented the public with the contention that young people must be truthfully and accurately educated about reproductive health as the best means of preventing venereal disease. With its stalwart affirmation of conventional religious beliefs, Stall's Self and Sex Series provided parents with aid in this novel responsibility and took part in an international conversation about the means of ensuring the health and well-being of future generations. The books anticipated the concerns that would form the agenda of the American Eugenics Society during the 1920s, while simultaneously tackling issues raised by the American Purity Alliance, which had held its first meeting in 1895.[25] Stall's work, then, kept an old-fashioned faith but tested the depths of new intellectual waters. Stall encouraged salespeople to connect the volumes with reforms promoting what was then cautiously referred to as personal purity, and what today would be called abstinence, for adolescents. His efforts were contested despite such delicacy, but he would survive assaults on his publishing empire while expanding the number of titles and authors who contributed to his success and to young people's guidance, promoting the key products of his publishing company until he died.

Under the direction of Stall; that of the succeeding copyright holder, his daughter, Frances C. Cash; and a board of directors that included her husband, the Self and Sex Series addressed male and female readers as they reached different stages of maturity, beginning with childhood and continuing through menopause, or in men's case, the age of forty-five.[26] Editions republished after Stall's death were promoted as "new" and "up-to-date," and deep blue covers replaced the once standard red.[27] Authorship was segregated for propriety's sake, with Stall writing books intended for male audiences and carefully selected female authors delivering advice to their own sex. The first of these women was Mary Wood-Allen. Wood-Allen's credentials included her training as a doctor, as well as her status as National Superintendent of the Purity Department of the Woman's Christian Temperance Union and as an author experienced in advising women on matters of hearth, home, and health.[28] She had, beginning in 1882, worked as a lecturer and writer whose subjects included sex education, only to encounter difficulties and resistance; eventually her perception of the importance of teaching "God's truth of generation" led her into independent publishing. This print project won her the notice of the WCTU leadership, and WCTU president Frances Willard's endorsement of the first book for girls in Stall's series, *What a Young Girl Ought to Know*. Throughout these activities, Wood-Allen's health was compromised, and her daughter remembered her dictating the content of the Vir books to a stenographer from her bed.[29]

Later, Wood-Allen would be joined in providing direction to female

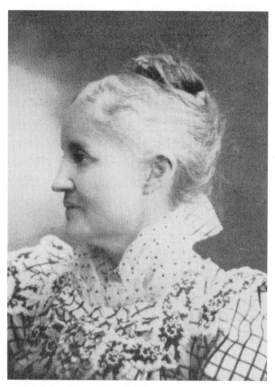

5. Physician Mary Wood-Allen was among the more popular and prolific writers of reproductive health information for female readers.—Kinsey Institute for Research in Sex, Gender, and Reproduction. Reproduced with permission.

readers by Emma Drake, a physician in Denver, Colorado. Stall presented Drake's selection as the result of a writing contest judged by a "committee of prominent ladies."[30] Her winning, though ultimately revised, manuscript became *What a Young Wife Ought to Know* (Wood-Allen had authored, in between these volumes, *What a Young Woman Ought to Know*). Stall had offered "a prize of $1,000 for best manuscript addressed to Young Wives," and when the book was published in 1901, he advertised it as the "$1,000 Prize Book, by Mrs. Emma F. A. Drake, M.D."—a strategy resembling an 1888 contest for sex education essays hosted by the Western Secretarial Institute.[31] Drake's and Wood-Allen's medical credentials legitimized Stall's endeavor, and by 1906, their leadership in the cause of social hygiene would be recognized with positions on the executive committee of the National Purity Conference.[32]

Announcements of new releases in the periodical press of the day indicate that *What a Young Boy Ought to Know* was the first title published in 1897, followed within a few months by *What a Young Girl Ought to Know,* and by *What a Young Man Ought to Know* just before the year's end.[33] Later Stall would describe his motivation for developing the rest of the series by saying he "was quick to recognize the leadings of Providence."[34] As even the first editions of these early titles bore complete lists of titles and authors, and the prominent individuals asked to provide pre-publication testimonials for *What a Young Boy Ought To Know* remarked not just on the single volume but on an anticipated set, Stall must have been quite quick indeed.[35] Reviews of the books he published, in conjunction with the content upon which writers commented, indicated contemporary responses to the novel features that Stall used in his bid for consumer attention.

Stall's books were full ones, typically featuring more than 200 pages of promotions, portraits, detailed tables of content, and lengthy chapters. The many pages of sometimes rather small print prompted one reviewer to describe an 1897 volume as "perhaps needlessly long," but it was still pronounced "admirable" and given the endorsement that "it may safely be commended to those for whom it was written."[36] Much as became the custom of other reformers interested in questions of reproductive health, Stall's books proffered one sort of advice to male readers and other ideas to female ones; this decision to emulate the practices of reformers, rather than the single-treatise approach largely extant in print culture, was significant and became the basis for another marketing claim that highlighted the difference between his books and those already on the market.

When Stall went to press with *What a Young Boy Ought to Know* in 1897, he did so with awareness of his entry into questionable legal terrain, his competition, and his status as a novice writer of hygiene literature. The preface to this first book explained its difference from nineteenth-century titles like Dr. John Harvey Kellogg's *Plain Facts For Old And Young,* which readers had kept in print for almost fifteen years: "We cannot but feel that the division of our subject into separate treatises, suited respectively in style and subject-matter to boys and men in different periods and conditions of life, will be found one of the best features which has ever been introduced to literature of this kind. The mistake of placing in the hands of a child a book containing information for grown persons is too obvious to need any discussion."[37] Thus a master of the genre was disarmed, and Stall marked himself as an innovator in a small but established area of publishing.[38] This remarkable argument discreetly voiced contemporary concerns about the nefarious effects of any sort of sexual content on impressionable young people. Among those whose word readers could count on to shore up Stall's confident self-assessment was Anthony Comstock. Stall printed the Secretary of the New York Society for the Suppression of Vice's photograph and his praise: "I hope it may be blessed to the elevation of the thoughts and hearts of the boys of this nation," he wrote of the series.[39] Stall would continue to use this endorsement years later when he found himself the target of his erstwhile supporter's investigations.

To most, the initial book was innocuous and even commendable. *What a Young Boy Ought to Know* began with the arrival of a baby sister, prompting a fictive young boy, Harry, to ask, "Where did Baby come from?" Stall, in a self-referential product placement, reminded readers that he published *Talks to the King's Children* and other books for young people: "The parents have turned to the author of Harry's books for an answer to Harry's question." Thus was born a new book, which, regardless of its title and his prior denunciations of generalist hygiene treatises, Stall maintained, "will be found equally interesting to both men and women, young and old."[40] The dramatic situation was furthered by references to new technology, as the text envisioned young Harry being allowed to listen to Stall's recorded voice. Only one reviewer ever remarked upon the device, seething with indignation that "the self-complacent nasal of the phonograph" could be used to "put prurient ideas" into the minds of "a gaping circle of enquiring youth."[41]

Stall thus launched an intricate account of the creation of the universe as a prelude to his discussion of human reproduction, a context that led *Ladies' Home Journal* editor Edward Bok to tell him, "you have compassed the whole subject."[42] This first book in the series established a rationale for a man of God to write about the science of sexual health, while hinting at a well-to-do, intelligent, and forward-thinking parent as part of its intended audience. It also rested upon belief in the divine and in "technological progress," a perspective subsequently critiqued by historian Carl Becker and later scholars as the "telos of American culture." Becker's comment that "the word Progress, like the Cross or the Crescent, is a symbol that stands for a social doctrine, a philosophy of human destiny" affords an apt description of Stall's print enterprise.[43]

Demonstrating the propriety of readers' reliance on reproductive health advice was fundamental to Stall's rhetorical and financial aims. *What a Young Boy Ought to Know* explained the approach that Stall wished his readers to bring to this subject: "Now we do not blush or regard it impure to study the wonderful wisdom and power which God displayed in the creation of Adam and Eve. Neither should we, when we think properly of the no less wonderful and mysterious manner in which God created Cain and Abel, their children, and in which He is still from day to day and year to year, raising up a new generation to take the places of their parents, when they shall have died and passed away." Alluding to biblical matters allowed Stall to proclaim procreation, which he recognized as a medical matter being advanced by the work of doctors like Alfred Fournier and Prince A. Morrow, a nonetheless "sacred subject."[44] He in turn popularized scientific knowledge of the body by nesting it in a devout philosophy of life on earth.

In spite of his firmly Creationist perspective, Stall's series steadfastly acknowledged contemporary science and technology, while distinguishing between the way God brought the world into being and the way recent inventions came to be. These messages attributed superior powers to God and lauded human accomplishments by giving them a divine provenance. The tributes to innovation were the prelude to discussions of reproduction that explained this complex subject as God's power at work in the world, a message subsequently endorsed by organizations from the U.S. Navy to the YMCA.

Human accomplishment, especially as manifested in recent technical feats, was thus a recurring theme in the Self and Sex Series. *What a Young Boy Ought to Know* rehearsed the recent invention of the locomotive, the steamship, the telegraph, and the telephone as the human use of God's gifts. Stall distinguished between organic and inorganic phenomena, concepts intrinsic to lessons on reproduction, because, as he explained to Harry, "To some of the works of His creation God has given the power to beget or produce others like themselves. Such objects learned men call organic objects" while others "are to abide until God shall destroy them, and hence it was not necessary that they should have given to them power to reproduce themselves."[45] Human beings, he stated, belonged to the first category. Stall thus portrayed reproduction as a God-given property nonetheless reconcilable with modern science. His authorship, and the work of his partners in the series, rested on these kinds of intricate connections between divine and scientific texts, promoting achievements in science and technology as emblematic of the attitudes his readers should adopt with regard to reproduction.

Female readers were to hold fast to notions of femininity and observe the way "Godlike" imagination produced poetry, art, and music.[46] While her daughter described Wood-Allen as a learned feminist whose difficult childhood gave her "insight into the duties and problems of motherhood," the books that Wood-Allen published with Stall expressed sentiment as often as science.[47] In *What a Young Girl Ought to Know*, girls were instructed in the benefits of public health, but Wood-Allen emphasized the unique nature of the female mind, body, and role in society and her home through sections of the book devoted to topics such as "Girls Sometimes Wish They Were Boys" and "The Influence of Girls on the Habits of Young Men." Differences between a girl's and a woman's body were discussed so that young girls knew to avoid the ways a woman might "tempt a man to do wrong."[48] In all this advice, Wood-Allen presented information as a means of preventing her readers from inadvertent harm, certain that they would choose right, which she equated with decorous behavior and attitudes, rather than the wrongs of bodily pleasure or personal freedom. Still, a faint echo of the scientific can be heard in her plea that girls should "read the lives of plants and flowers as they grow in the garden, read the experiences of the birds in the trees. . . . To be interested in home duties and in nature is the safest pleasure for the young girl."[49] This sort of caution, written as Fournier published mounting evidence of the contagious and still incurable aspects of syphilis, reinforced domestic ideals of womanhood, but its repressive messages were not unrelated to the real, and in some respects darkening, world.

In this context, nature represented an opportunity for people to observe God's intentions at work in the world and to model their own conduct accordingly. One passage in *What a Young Boy Ought to Know* urged that readers learn from birds not only the basics of an egg's development into a hatchling but also ordained parental and spousal roles. Stall characterized nesting as a loving and instinctive process: "You will have noticed that the mamma bird prefers to sit most of the time on the eggs and keep them warm, but all the while the papa bird has stayed close by, coming often to sit on a branch near the nest, and chirp and sing, and thus cheer and keep the mamma bird company." This anthropomorphic reasoning was carried still further, lest his lessons from nature strike readers as too matter-of-fact: "At times, when the mamma bird was tired, they would both fly away together, and after a few moments, the papa bird would hurry back to take the mamma bird's place, and keep the eggs warm and guard them from harm, while the mamma bird would take such rest and recreation as she needed or wished. The home life of two such parent birds is devoted and sweet, and no man or boy can watch it without learning from the birds lessons of love and fidelity."[50] Stall moved from his avian model of domestic bliss to a terrain simultaneously more traditional and more scientific.

His ideals of involved parenting aside, Stall saw men and women's lives in gendered terms. Woman, he told young readers, depended on her husband to protect her "not only from outward physical danger, but every impurity of thought, word, and deed."[51] In these safe, even sanctimonious counsels, Stall engaged the themes of Progressive reform by encouraging readers to respond to new social problems—the licentiousness of urban environments and rising divorce rates among them—with naturally old-fashioned values.

The birds were Stall's segue into human reproduction, and he turned from this fanciful veneration of nature to more medical explanations. He told readers about the existence of microscopic organisms, identifying the function of ova, sperm, and semen before eclipsing this discussion with the explanation that "in the state of pure and holy marriage, God has ordained that the ovum shall be fertilized by the requisite and proper bodily contact of the husband."[52] This naming of at least some parts was far more technical and specific than much printed information available to the ordinary reader on the cusp of the twentieth century. A decade after Stall produced the first edition of *What a Young Boy Ought to Know*, reformers still decried young people's lack of information about reproduction, attributing a high proportion of out-of-wedlock pregnancies to ignorance.[53] Stall's modest account of the sex act, constrained though it was, advanced the level of accurate knowledge of the human body available to preteens and adolescents.

The Vir books written specifically for girls and young women sometimes lacked even this relative frankness in their accounts of pregnancy and birth. *What a Young Girl Ought to Know* emphasized maternal love for the baby that would be born, and in doing so conformed to guidance that later doctors declared a girl's prerogative—instruction in "the function and sacredness of motherhood."[54] Wood-Allen described gestation as the time that "the young" were "kept within the mother's body."[55] She would also acknowledge the process of labor, writing elsewhere, "the door of your little room opened with much pain and suffering to me, and then you came into the world."[56] From this proximity to medical fact, Wood-Allen returned to the rosy glow of maternity, depicting a mother's rapturous enthrallment with her newborn. In *What a Young Woman Ought to Know*, she approached the matter in terms both direct and delicate. Wood-Allen established "the fact of sex" for her readers, but left them to understand it as "the expression of the whole nature, through the physical" and "the vital creative force endeavoring to reach a tangible result." She cautioned, "Holy in its inception, it can be degraded to the vilest uses."[57] From this veiled discussion, Wood-Allen turned to topics such as "The Law of Heredity" and "The Effects of Immorality on the Race."

Elsewhere in her pages for young women, however, Wood-Allen acknowledged sexual desire more openly, hoping to constrain youthful passion. She lectured young women against flirting and allowing themselves to be kissed by young men, reporting overheard conversations among fellows who shared their assessments of the young women who permitted, as Wood-Allen termed it, familiarities. Being talked of in this way, she was certain, was something no female reader would want. She also wrote against romance novels whose "sentimental fancies" could cause readers to become "unduly stimulated and aroused."[58] Yet even as she cautioned against sexual excitement, she was explicit about how it occurred, recognizing it as a temptation for girls as well as boys: "The stimulation of the sex organs is accompanied with a pleasurable sensation, and this excitement may be created by mechanical means, or even by thought."[59] To dissuade young women from such forms of pleasure, she labeled masturbation illicit and harmful, dwelling on readers' potential to feel shame and fear the consequent ruin of "the complexion" and destruction of "mental power and memory." Wood-Allen did not, however, condemn her readers to joyless lives; she encouraged them to take their pleasures elsewhere, noting that "every normal function of the body is attended with a pleasurable sensation."[60] Although members of the American Society for Sanitary and Moral Prophylaxis criticized the books as more prurient than practical and Wood-Allen once had difficulty finding a publisher for work, this blend of medical perspective and motherly admonishments won praise from reviewers.[61] She was credited with presenting "a simple, direct statement of the value of health and the way to preserve it . . . told distinctly, but with refinement."[62]

Similarly, Stall's thinking about sexuality did not diverge far from his religious colleagues' views, and these ideas were generally congruent with much late nineteenth-century medical wisdom. Writing at the same time that Havelock Ellis attempted to revise Victorian strictures against masturbation, Stall condemned the practice as a health threat to both the individual and his future children, identifying masturbation both by this less judgmental term as well as the more contemporary labels of solitary vice and self-pollution.[63] He acknowledged that the act would result in pleasure, albeit temporarily, he wrote, relative to its inevitable, woeful consequences. He emphasized cleanliness via instruction on the importance of circumcision and instructions for cleaning intimate parts of the body.[64] It was perhaps this sort of lesson that led one reviewer of a later edition to urge "that when a boy has once read it he be instructed to burn it and not preserve it for future reference and reading."[65] For the most part, though, reviewers were less dramatic in their commentary, praising Stall as someone who "in no case . . . overstepped the bounds of the essential" or included "a word that could stimulate a morbid curiosity."[66] In their judgment, the series' medical and spiritual advice on sexuality was sound.

Wood-Allen and Stall went further than many dared at this time, by bringing syphilis to their readers' attention. That their efforts were not universally approved is unsurprising given dissent within the medical community about the disease's etiology. Wood-Allen named the disease and its effects, linking them to "an impure life" rather than, as Stall did, to "the germs of syphilis."[67] Syphilis, female readers were warned, "is practically incurable"; they were given the essence of Fournier's findings when told that this disease "may temporarily disappear, only to reappear in some other form later in life."[68] Yet Wood-Allen hinted in a footnote where more information was to be found, referring her reader to three chapters in *What Every Young Man Ought to Know* that explained "Evils to Be Shunned and Consequences to Be Dreaded" or venereal disease. Here Stall cited his conversations with physicians, reading of the medical literature, visits to hospitals and the Medical Museum of Anatomy in the nation's capital, and acquaintance "with some persons who have suffered from these fearful diseases," insisting that "it was through them that my attention was first called to a thoughtful consideration and study of their terrible effects."[69] It was not for such content but for his marketing practices that the books drew flak. It was the reading of material intended for the opposite sex, as Wood-Allen suggested, that some found disturbing, and one doctor who observed young men purchasing *What a Young Woman Ought to Know* on the college campus where he taught called their behavior "demoralizing and degrading."[70]

In most circles, however, the potential affliction of the innocent warranted what under other circumstances would have been outrageous speech. Stall wrote, "Outside the medical profession there is general and almost profound ignorance concerning the prevalence, character and sad consequences of the diseases which afflict those who are given to illicit and unlawful sexual indulgence." This complaint commonly served his contemporaries as a justification for broaching sensitive health topics, and Stall reinforced it with appeals to conservative medical expertise. Some few physicians clung to the idea that transmission of syphilis within a family was evidence of "the inscrutable law of God, which decrees that the sins of the father shall be visited upon the children," and Stall quoted them authoritatively, even if he did not believe in this principle absolutely.[71] While his sense of Christian dogma was unrelenting and he insisted on abstinence and efforts to prevent nocturnal emissions, he would not condemn the desperately ill to lives of unaided suffering. Like Morrow and those who formed the American Society for Sanitary and Moral Prophylaxis, Stall thought syphilis and gonorrhea were concentrated in cities, particularly among the young adults who moved there to find work. The transition to adulthood, with its presumed interest in sexual activity, then, was a significant theme in the Self and Sex Series, and here as well Stall showed his familiarity with recent research.

Because Stall understood adolescence as spanning ages fourteen through twenty-five, multiple volumes addressed the concerns of this cohort. All his books differentiated between puberty, as the series of physical changes experienced during the late teen years, and adolescence. The preliminary physical and emotional changes were first referred to in *What a Young Boy Ought to Know,* with a chapter that focused on "The Passage from Infancy to Manhood." Parallel ideas appeared in the books for female readers. Stall catalogued new bodily attributes, from bones to voices. In an apparent echo of Fournier, he explained, "The sexual parts begin to develop, and . . . [he] becomes the subject of new sensations and desires, which he is not able to interpret or comprehend."[72] Awakening sexuality was inscribed as an essential component of adolescence.

Stall singled out the ages between fourteen and eighteen as the "most trying" ones. He focused on behaviors that subsequently would become stereotypes of adolescence, emphasizing teens' "contrariness" and "rebellion." His sympathies seemed to lie with these troubled creatures, as he counseled parents who "do not understand their condition, and who have forgotten their own feelings and experiences when at the same age" about how to ease a young person's transition to maturity. Significantly, in this discussion Stall mentioned the German psychological theory of "storm and stress" as an essential characteristic of adolescence.[73]

His use of this phrase is one more indication that he consulted the most current scholarship on the subjects about which he wrote. Even the first editions of *What a Young Boy Ought to Know* included this now familiar reference to the turbulence popularly associated with adolescence, reflecting Stall's connection to others grappling with the problems of youth and health. G. Stanley Hall, whose monumental 1904 publication *Adolescence* marked the beginning of adolescent psychology, credited the "storm and stress" theory with vast explanatory power. Hall was a member of Purity Movement associations and believed in the need "for plainer talk" about reproductive health with young people.[74] Stall moved in these same circles, and his reliance on Hall's introduction of this phrase to American readers indicates the seriousness of his efforts to understand adolescent well-being. This reliance on recent ground-breaking research encouraged contemporary readers to see the books as credible treatments of pressing present concerns.

Selling the Self and Sex Series Near and Far

Stall's marketing, as much as the content of his titles, distinguished them from competing publications, and Stall promoted the uniqueness and the success of his approach to sex education alike. Evidence of an increasing readership was itself a testimonial to potential readers, whom he and his staff were ever ready to court. Stall recruited a door-to-door sales force that he guided via a book of their own called *The Successful Selling of the Self and Sex Series.*[75] Printed in 1907, the 300-plus-page book described sales pitches, identified likely readers—or at least purchasers—and indicated the importance of collecting debts. Later, Stall supplemented this resource with a free serial that reached many in the book trade, a "little house organ . . . which we mail

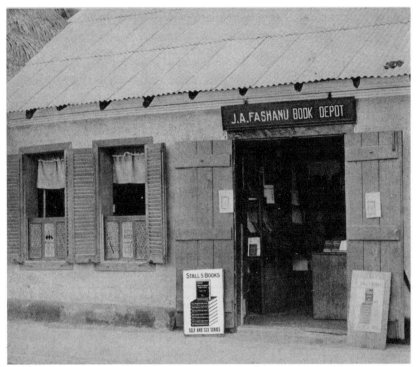

6. Publisher and minister Sylvanus Stall encouraged door-to-door salespeople and retailers to share the means by which they attracted readers' attention to his books, and many responded to his call for marketing ideas. General Research Division, The New York Public Library, Astor, Lenox and Tilden Foundations. Reproduced with permission.

to each member of the selling force in the various book shops, not only to familiarize themselves with the selling qualities of our own publications, but to inspire them to sell other books worth while and to make them more efficient as salesmen," as its editor L. M. Cross explained.[76]

Cross promoted Vir titles, interviewed publishers and salespeople, suggested service strategies, and documented trends in publishing and world events. He and Stall traveled together, assessing sales of Vir titles across the country and around the world. Cross profiled the book people they met and the stores they visited in the company's new publication from 1911 until his death in 1928.[77] News of individuals' marriages and illnesses, aphorisms, and even an account of the time

Cross's son spent fighting in Europe during World War I also filled its pages. A short, secondary instructional work, "How to Make Good as a Book Salesman," was also advertised in *Successful Selling,* as were occasional training seminars.[78]

In these manuals, Stall revealed the means of moving sex education from private conversation to purchased text in the early twentieth century. He urged his employees to use the books themselves, the contemporary social concern with social hygiene, and the strategic dialogues with which he supplied them to make sales. While reviewers shared their intense convictions that these titles would help parents who struggled with task of telling their children about sex, a dialogue doctors argued was newly essential to stemming the endemic spread of syphilis and gonorrhea, Stall emphasized how to bring about sales. Although he frequently drew attention to the religious and philanthropic nature of social hygiene work and aligned Vir Publishing with this cause, he also exploited readers' religious values and aspirational ideals in order to sell the Self and Sex Series.

The late Victorian and early Progressive Era Purity Movement was fundamental to Stall's marketing of the series. Chastity prior to monogamous marriage was a recurrent theme in his treatises and in the concerns of this reform community. Purity advocates encouraged sexual restraint for young men and women alike, and most salutary works considered the cumulative effects of a young person's many activities, reading habits among them, on his or her sexual health. Those who focused attention on social hygiene and youthful purity urgently declaimed the need for "innocence not ignorance." Stall's directions to his staff invoked the same values, yet were strident about the financial consequences of failing to spur readers to place his books in their home libraries.

Making a sale, Stall, explained, involved addressing a simple problem: Potential buyers wanted to keep their money, while salespeople wanted to part them from it. To resolve this dilemma, Stall assured his employees, a canvasser must bring about in the buyer's "mind a desire for your books which shall exceed the desire which he has for his dollars." Moving the individual toward this perspective meant convincing him or her that "whatever value the individual places on happiness, blessing, prosperity, and health, that is the value of the book which is best suited to his need." Stall told his canvassers that sales depended on their skillful execution of three core behaviors: "securing a hearing," "creating the desire," and "obtaining the subscription." The odds of succeeding in these steps were improved, he assured them, by knowing the books they sold. Having acknowledged earlier that both men and women were equally suited to sales careers, he directed that "each day before the canvasser starts out he should read a chapter in one or other of the books, and thus return daily to his work with renewed information and enthusiasm." It was not enough to be versed in Stall's ideas; the physical condition of the book had to be well handled, but not overly worn, to be persuasive. In a section titled "Working the Book" Stall explained how to treat a demonstration copy so "that it will fall open at any desired page or paragraph" that might be needed in testifying to the book's merits.[79]

No detail was too insignificant for Stall's attention, and he seemed convinced that canvassers would peruse his instructions with the same deliberation and care that he had taken in preparing this guidance. He admonished sales people to be careful about eye contact and not to memorize a sales pitch lest this practice result in a "sing song and unnatural tone of voice" whose manner would strike listeners as "parrot-like." He described ways to glean a homeowner's name and other descriptive details from a neighbor, in order to adapt one's approach at the next door, as well as how to walk through a neighborhood in ways that would disarm suspicions that the salesperson was merely "some peddler." Personal hygiene was also discussed, as Stall informed his staff that it would be difficult to sell The Self and Sex titles if their own appearance suggested they had not profited from the books' advice.[80]

In tandem with his aggressive focus on sales, Stall repeatedly assured canvassers that their purpose was a noble one: "In view of the fact that we are prosecuting a great crusade for personal and social purity . . . it is proper for the canvasser to present himself in the light of one who is prosecuting the work of a special crusade." He regarded the salesperson as the minister's "coworker" and encouraged those who confronted a reluctant buyer to believe "You are this person's benefactor. Intellectually, physically, socially this person is measurably famished.

He or she is suffering for lack of the very information these books contain." Refusal, then, meant not that the individual did not to want or need the book, only that its benefits were not understood by someone whose judgment was clouded by lack of knowledge. Anticipating the sorts of discouragement a canvasser might face at a time when sex was controversial yet increasingly in the public eye, Stall told his staff to "fix clearly in your mind wherein these books differ from any other books upon the subject of sex ever written."[81] The series' connection to contemporary reform shored up salespeople's doubts, then, as well as hesitant purchasers' concerns about the value of the Self and Sex Series.

As was conventional among hygiene reformers and, before them, the colporteurs of the American Tract Society, Stall was mindful of the role of books and reading in young people's lives.[82] While he and his authors warned young people that inappropriate reading threatened their personal purity, he told canvassers how they might use this same activity to sway parents who hesitated to buy his titles for their children. He contended, "Generally some boy or girl is known through the neighborhood as a great reader. If you know that fact you can always make capital out of it, as it is quite a compliment to have you speak about it." He cautioned, "Of course you must do it tactfully." Mothers, Stall observed, were most likely to succumb to this kind of flattery.[83] Elsewhere, though, he suggested that canvassers deflect attention from his books, emphasizing their ideals rather than their material form to skeptics. He modeled a response to those who suggested Vir's representatives were simply salespeople and its books merely another commodity: "You cannot class me as a book agent for I am engaged in a great campaign which is being extensively waged for personal and social purity." Implicit in this appeal was the assertion that the series, in contrast to less costly popular literature, provided safe reading matter for young people. The value ascribed to reading in this mercantile campaign, then, shifted to reflect ranging social perceptions about the dangers and the importance of literacy, but its protean character was always to the seller's advantage.

Stall's prevarications supported his aim of selling books and recognized the inevitable difficulties that a salesperson would confront.

An extensive portion of *The Successful Selling of the Self and Sex Series* responded to the myriad refusals that might be encountered at a stranger's door in an unfamiliar town, whether the target contended that "I haven't time to read," "We can get all the books we want in the public library," or even "The crops are a failure." These "Canvasser's Formulas" relentlessly challenged the notion that people might be unable to afford books. Stall counseled canvassers that "the cry of 'hard times' is heard at all times" and that they might try "ignoring, evading, and treating lightly" before "treating seriously" any refusal made on economic grounds.[84] The publisher reasoned that appeals to the ideal of self-improvement was the basis for a calculated, practiced refutation of a buyer's rebuff:

> Some of the most appreciative letters we have ever received at the office of publication have come from just such homes of poverty. Women who scrubbed and washed, have written to tell us that they would sooner deny their children a bag of flour, than to have denied them the benefits and blessings which they secured from the reading of *What a Young Boy Ought to Know* and *What a Young Girl Ought to Know,* and from the books to young men and young women. We appeal to both your sense and your sentiment. If these books are a benefaction and a blessing to humanity then their benefits cannot be denied to the poor without doing them great wrong. . . . They need these books, and these books will be a blessing to them in every way, and it is your duty to make them appreciate this fact. You do them a great injustice if you think they are too poor to purchase.[85]

Stall's contention that books meant more than food was not original, as Wood-Allen's daughter also told a story about the time her mother presented the children with books rather than a Thanksgiving dinner, promising them that "you'll never miss the turkey when you read this book."[86] Stall also mentioned the names of famous men from impoverished backgrounds, Abraham Lincoln among them, whose examples might encourage a purchase, because "it was helpful books that lifted these boys to places of eminence." Neither the poor nor those who had failed to live according to Stall's notions of moral purity could afford to be without these books, he argued. He identified the "hired man and hired girl" as yielding recipients of such messages, noting, "You will sell to most of them."[87] He seemed oblivious to the mercenary aspect of his directions, perhaps believing that his tone simply echoed the encouraging narratives shared by ATS members.[88] Colporteurs sought doorstep conversions; Stall, however, wanted cash.

The subsequent overview of the laws of credit and the necessity of collecting debts only heightened the impression that Stall's most fervent feeling was for his income. He described surety bonds that guaranteed payment by leveraging the value of one's home, the need to have a judge as a witness to enforce certain types of contracts, and other legal mechanisms for assuring payment. Canvassers were warned that they, too, were obligated to Vir Publishing for the cost of volumes that they distributed. That salespeople worked for Stall under the cloud of such inducements suggests either his products, his appeals, or the two in combination were persuasive indeed.

Stall's employees responded faithfully to his dictates and his insistence on their involvement in discovering means of making sales. He seemed attuned to every venue where a would-be book buyer might be found, but his awareness of these opportunities was not exclusively his own. Stall recognized that canvassers' accounts of their experiences on the road might help others improve their abilities to sign subscribers. He directed the salesperson to share "any personal method which he adopts with special success." "Send us both sunshine and shadow," he wrote. These reports, in turn, allowed Stall to regale new or discouraged salespeople with the activities of those who succeeded, as one enterprising individual did, in seeing a volume purchased by all the members of a young men's Christian reading group or an exemplary canvasser whose sales in the Allegheny region of New York and Pennsylvania resulted, on the average, to "about one copy to each ten inhabitants, counting men, women and children."[89]

It is unclear, then, whether his insistence that if a canvasser's knock at the front door was not answered, calling at the kitchen door, where a potentially pliable servant girl would answer, was the fruit of his own bookselling experience or an inference gleaned from his employees. He advised sellers to call on preachers upon arrival in a new town, to seek the minister's sanction and even an announcement about the series from the pulpit. He advised, though, against making one's first sale to the minister, who might depress the local market by lending the newly acquired volumes to his congregation. Stall suggested placing ads in local newspapers and offered prepared copy for these announcements. He instructed his sales staff to contact the Young Men's Christian Association and other like-minded organizations that might furnish local membership lists, particularly names of those enrolled in Bible study classes, thereby identifying potential targets.[90]

These tactics were only part of Stall's extensive battery of sales techniques. Despite this attention to enhancing the productivity of Vir Publishing canvassers, bookstores began to stock these volumes around 1910. Stall communicated with stores directly and through the newly created periodical that came to be known as *Successful Selling*. Where the monograph *Successful Selling of the Self and Sex Series* was written for an internal audience, the new, square-shaped magazine, which averaged between 20 and 32 pages per issue, reached multitudes of people involved in the business of publishing and selling books.[91] True to its title, the periodical carried ads for the Self and Sex Series and explained Stall's successes, so that readers learned that 1914 and 1920 were years that saw some of the strongest sales in the company's history.[92] News of the first two price increases in 1920 that pushed the dollar cost of a single title to $1.20 and then to $1.30 were softened by promises of continuing "generous discounts" to retail sellers.[93] Incentives and advice alike, then, filled the pages of the new Vir endeavor.

The magazine also proposed means by which sellers could improve their own profits. A brief filler following the justification of price increases guaranteed, "A window publicity of Stall's Books is sure to bring increased sales." Bookstore windows with displays of Stall's books were featured regularly in *Successful Selling*, implying that booksellers need not be ashamed to acknowledge their stock of hygiene titles. One such photograph was accompanied by a note from the manager of the American Baptist Publication Society store, who called its promotional display of the Self and Sex Series "one of the best window displays we have ever made," because "it has proved satisfactory in the way of sales, and in making our windows unusually attractive."[94] Another window banner informed shoppers that "Stall's Books on Avoided Subjects" were in their "Third Million Edition."[95]

The series' much-touted acquisition of "two thousand new readers daily" also stemmed from Stall's involvement with Christian missionary societies that sent his volumes overseas. Stall claimed that this foreign dissemination was "unsolicited" by Vir Publishing, the result instead of requests for "the privilege to translate."[96] This distribution of the Self and Sex Series suggests that at least prior to World War II, different conditions antedated Beth Luey's findings that in international publishing, "decisions are made by buyers rather than sellers" and that works with culturally incompatible messages "are unlikely to be translated."[97] Stall proudly indicated that volumes were sent overseas by missionaries who relied on the advice manuals to instruct converts in the tenets of pure living. "Evangelists, purity lecturers and public speakers . . . have commended them from the platform to multitudes of people in every part of the world," he wrote.[98] A number of organizations, then, created audiences for Stall's treatises. He operated years in advance of the UNESCO *Index Translatorium,* so assessing the reach of his titles can be done only through marketing materials and articles on translation and dissemination efforts.

Translation and publication rights outside the United States became significant, though English-language copies were sold in other countries. Stall's account of how many languages his works were distributed in varied with the source in which he announced the endeavors—ranging from as few as six to as many as fourteen—but he readily identified his associates. The Church Missionary Societies of America and England were prominent among them, sending copies to Korea and many other countries.[99] The YMCA's efforts were also significant, at least from the publisher's perspective. Stall reported that this group alone sent 10,000 copies to India, China, and Japan, although YMCA narratives of its overseas work fail to acknowledge the distribution of Stall's titles among their efforts, emphasizing their self-published titles instead.[100] Secondary publishers included the Rev. A. Jewson in Calcutta, the Christian Literature Society for India in Madras, and the Methodist Publishing House in Tokyo, the last described in a contem-

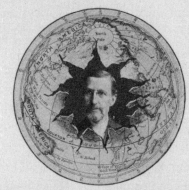
7. In a bid to demonstrate the merits of his titles, Sylvanus Stall promoted the worldwide audiences for his Self and Sex Series. General Research Division, The New York Public Library, Astor, Lenox and Tilden Foundations. Reproduced with permission.

porary magazine article as "the largest Christian publishing house in Japan."[101]

These connections, however, were not without their strains. In 1900, the Japanese translations of titles for male readers were begun, it was reported, "to counteract vices so common in that country." Those responsible for this work, however, were forced to confront "the fact that the Japanese language contains no words to convey the thought that has been unfolded in such a unique manner in this deservedly popular series of books issued by the Vir Publishing Company of Philadelphia."[102] Despite such setbacks, Stall contended that the series met "a universal need" and was "suited to all races, to all nations, to all classes, and to all conditions of men and women."[103] Building an international print empire, rather than cultural sensitivity, marked his success.

While Asian-language translations bolstered missionaries' attempts to convince converts to adopt Western religious values and cultural practices, straightforward financial motives seemed to spur the production of European-language editions. Initially, Stall indicated the availability of French editions via a Swiss publishing house, as well as the existence of Spanish, Swedish, and German presses. Dutch editions were brought out in both Holland and South Africa. Shortly before his death, Stall boasted, "In France, Germany, Russia, Holland, Italy, Spain, Sweden and other countries marked on the map of Europe, the people are reading [the books'] informing and clean messages in their own tongue."[104] Ads of this era acknowledged the war being fought on the Continent, while Vir Publishing conducted a steady English-language business in the United Kingdom, with a London office headed by Charles R. King, whose sale of "more than half a million of our various publications" was attributed to his reliance on good advertising and prompt service.[105] Of all the translations, only the European-language editions were made available within the United States, though Stall instructed canvassers to downplay the availability of non-English titles within this country. The matter of language, then, both enhanced and checked Stall's marketing.

These distinctive efforts spawned a print industry that eventually sprawled around the globe and across the years. The prominence of the Self and Sex Series reflected Stall's relentless self-promotion and his ability to respond to largely unmet, intensely private concerns about sex and the body at a time when many experts suggested there was much to fear and little to know beyond fear itself. His promotional strategies prompted individuals' purchase of informational texts on subjects very recently regarded as the exclusive province of physicians, when treated wholesomely, and the murky terrain of pornographers when not. Vir's books sold briskly throughout the nation and saw further dissemination across the globe in part because of awareness of their availability and assurances that their content was chaste rather than tawdry. *The Successful Selling of the Self and Sex Series*, then, was an apt description of Stall's enterprise, which opened markets for others who aspired to advise readers on the new rules of hygiene, as well as the title of Vir Publishing's training manual.

As the Self and Sex series thrived, others adopted and adapted Stall's distinctive agenda by producing their own social hygiene books in hopes that something like his prolific sales figures would become theirs, too. Stall and his international Vir Publishing Company were never alone in the rather remarkable enterprise of selling sexual health information during an era that, for all its technological and scientific advances, still evinced conservative social mores, and Stall surveyed the publishing industry vigilantly for cues about the status of the Self and Sex Series relative to its competition. His attention to the fluctuating number of medical and hygiene titles, as well as the way these works figured in the overall American book market, was one element of this awareness.[106] Stall understood that both physicians and publishers challenged his self-proclaimed status as the field's leader, and he recognized that tributes to Vir's approach to sex education, however sincere and well placed, would not preserve his empire. In its house publication, Vir belittled the contenders. Characterizing competing titles as "silly, weak imitations," Cross related an anonymous anecdote of a "prominent bookman" who dismissed the company's rivals as thieving copycats, saying, "All the good that is in some of them has been stolen from Stall's Books."[107] Such jibes did not dissuade the competition. Nonetheless, in the decades that followed, it was Stall's work that lingered in the public imagination.

Publishers like Haldeman-Julius, which later created the Little Blue Notebook series in Kansas, would echo Stall's familiar titles but not his religious dictates.[108] These presses operated under fewer restrictions than Stall had as he established his brand and his books in the late nineteenth century. Comstock-inspired censorship had waned—but not disappeared—with the anti-vice crusader's death in 1915. In 1918, a court ruling had decriminalized the use of condoms as a means of preventing sexually transmitted disease.[109] Further, the intervening years had seen innovations in the treatment of syphilis. A changed climate prevailed then, when William J. Fielding heralded a new era for female readers and began to depict Stall's books as even more intensely conservative than they were, announcing that one no longer lived when "*Every Young Woman* was not supposed to know much." In the 1920s, Fielding claimed, "Sex Phenomena" were "the very foundation of life, health and happiness." He provided female readers with diagrams of their internal and external reproductive anatomy, and while the clitoris was not identified pictorially, there was no sense of hesitancy or shame in his description, some pages later, of that organ as "plentifully supplied with nerves" and "the principal point of excitement in the female genitals."[110]

Strictures against reading were forgotten, replaced by a bold assertion in Fielding's chapter on adolescence that "the reading matter now in demand is stories and novels of romance, wherein she can peruse the love epistles of people who are acting the thoughts she feels and fulfill the pictures of her reveries; and of course, she identifies herself with the heroine."[111] The Little Blue Notebooks did not simply take advantage of the evocative phrasing that Stall had crafted and promoted over the years; the authors of these slim, pale blue pamphlets simultaneously used his long-standing works as a foil for their own commercially produced messages. Diminished, too, were Stall's teleological notions; instead, progress was represented by the unrestrained tone of these publications, their refusal to subordinate their health messages to religious lessons about morality and science.

That competitors discarded the minister's earnest and cautious warnings about sex did not mean the end of Stall's empire. Posthumous editions of his books perpetuated his reserved approach to sex information but emulated the day's slang to show their currency. The 1928 edition of *What a Young Husband Ought to Know,* dedicated to "the young husband who aims to be the pal and companion of the ideal girl who has become his partner in life," struck a freer tone than earlier commendations to "the young men who should be pure and strong."[112] Despite this linguistic emulation of '20s vogue, Self and Sex titles maintained a perspective on sexuality best regarded as nostalgic, and bookstores replaced the traveling salesperson's doorstep appeals. In this way Vir Publishing continued to sell the Self and Sex Series until 1937, when Thomas J. Parran Jr., director of the U.S. Public Health Service, declared a national campaign "against the scourge of syphilis," sanctioning public statements about sexual and reproductive health.[113]

For nearly forty years, Stall's works had persisted in popularizing information and ideas about reproductive health. He justified his entry into such questionable terrain by interlacing medical material with sentimental and sensational religious appeals for chastity. Thus leavened, the books in the Self and Sex Series connected readers with the ideas of doctors and reformers themselves at work around the world. In Stall's wake, others saw market opportunities where there once were sanctions against even relatively open communication about sex and diseases transmitted by intimate contact. Despite their sometimes appreciably more liberal content, succeeding publishers nonetheless hoped to capitalize on what this one-time Lutheran minister had helped to realize—modestly packaged and strategically promoted, popular sex information in America sold. In the short term, however, the demand for hygiene texts complicated the production of these materials at the very moment when they seemed poised to offer much—whether affluence, influence, or information—to so many people.

CHAPTER 5

BATTLING BOOKS

Censorship, Conservatism, and Market Competition

*Parents are beginning to realize the necessity of early instruction in
matters of sex. The social diseases, a few years ago a forbidden discussion, are receiving the consideration of many thoughtful citizens. The
public believes more than ever before that modern hygienic methods
should be applied to all communicable diseases.*

—F. N. WHITTIER

Even as humanitarian and opportunistic impulses shaped the distinctive print culture of Progressive Era hygiene literature, equally forceful
voices countered the aspirations of the genre's progenitors. The best-
known hygiene titles for young readers realized significant circulation
in the early twentieth century, and the realities of a growing market
inspired imitators as well as opponents of sharing real knowledge about
reproduction with adolescents. Challenges to hygiene titles emerged
from outside the industry and within. Paul S. Boyer has aptly noted that
when considered in its cultural context, "censorship history became
considerably more complex and less black and white."[1] The related
early twentieth-century phenomena of the success and the suppression
of hygiene texts were also complicated, consequential developments.

Although they never made best-seller lists, a number of titles nonetheless achieved significant circulations. Interest in sexual health texts
was documented primarily by publishers themselves. Sylvanus Stall's
boasts that many thousands of readers owned *What a Young Man
Ought to Know* or its companion volumes, along with equally self-con-
scious title-page counts of the imprints of not-for-profit texts, marked
the demand for sexual and reproductive health materials informed,
however speciously, by recent medical thinking. These self-generated
reports testified that the re-invigorated genre was attracting readers,
fostering competition, proprietary claims, and serious re-evaluations
of what constituted propriety in print. An endeavor that had begun

with declarations of the public interest, professional admiration, and good intentions was transformed as new figures joined the commercial fray and established writers reconsidered their roles and their responsibilities in assuring the common good. Initial, idealistic expectations about venereal disease prevention tracts shifted before seminal texts—works like Stall's first titles and Alfred Fournier's *Pour nos fils*—had been in print for even a decade.

Where a treatise's reach had once been all that mattered, the ownership of words and the presumed ability to profit from them or to protect them increasingly became an issue. Whether motivated by monetary or medical aims, writers did not assume that their initial popular works would tell adolescents all they ought to know. Instead, a succession of new books was designed to appeal to previous purchasers and new audiences alike. This authorial activity, sparked by the evolving scientific investigation of disease and the once little expected but continually more voluminous reading and redistribution practices, also reflected a largely unacknowledged competition. The demonstrable consumption of credible, current health information likewise reduced authors' willingness to participate in the networks that Fournier had instigated to share free, uncopyrighted texts. Even physicians, whose professional ethics prohibited advertising cures for specific ailments and self-promotion, began to distinguish between the objects of these restrictions and their writerly endeavors.[2]

Three authors' later texts called attention to these dynamics and their entailments. Fournier's secondary, treatment-oriented writings were not affiliated with the French Society for Sanitary and Moral Prophylaxis, which sponsored the printing of his first text for young men and supported its distribution abroad; conversely, Stall's independent publication of *The Social Peril* revealed his connections to other prominent American figures invested in educating young people about sexual health. A third writer and physician, Winfield Scott Hall, indicated his understanding of these two men's achievements in his efforts to emulate their success. Each writer's work signaled different dimensions of the shifting profile of sexual health texts for young people.

Shortly before the release of Fournier's later guidance, Stall also shared more specific contemporary medical knowledge about venereal disease in *The Social Peril,* a stand-alone, full-length work published by Vir in 1905. While the provocative title resonated with the concerns that characterized the Self and Sex Series, its reception diverged sharply from that of Stall's previous titles. Instead, physician Prince A. Morrow questioned his right to share medical messages with a general readership. Stall was confronted not just by high-minded organizers like Morrow but also, less directly, by Winfield Scott Hall. A conservative reformer, Hall wrote and published over the course of many years, eventually crafting messages to show young people the urgency of protecting their reproductive health through sexual restraint. His myriad works included *Instead of Wild Oats: A Little Book for the Youth of 18 and Over* and *Sexual Knowledge: The Knowledge of the Self and Sex in Simple Language.* In these titles, Hall turned his credentials to competing for Stall's readers. Together, these subsequent books demonstrated that the emerging demand for hygiene texts could create difficulties at least as challenging as the ones that had beset their novelty.

The newer treatises by Fournier, whose turn-of-the-century booklets had launched this textual movement, and by Stall, whose commercialization of hygiene books helped to swell the global market for such work, reflected subtle though significant changes in writing about sexual health, even as Hall trod in the footsteps of so many previous efforts to inform young people about venereal disease. These volumes indicated that members of the medical profession actively pursued both remedies for sexually transmitted infection and authorial revenue; yet they operated simultaneously with reformers and authorities whose defense of public decency was not modified by awareness of sexual health as a public health concern. Boyer had indicated that "the branch of Progressive reform most sympathetic to the vice-society movement was that most concerned with sexual morality"; yet the complexities of threatened censorship and attempted publication defy such easy generalization.[3]

The Social Peril provoked further demonstrations of authors' attempts to control public access to their expertise and forced Stall to fend off allegations of impropriety. Although he preemptively pursued endorsements to demonstrate that his books offered modest counsel to young people and their parents, his strategy won readers but failed to ward off other challenges. His 1905 text, *The Social Peril,* became the target of investigations. Because laws as well professional conventions governed publications, a prominent, if skeptical, First Amendment attorney came to play a role in resolving the conflicts over rights and decency in print. Theodore Schroeder, a nonconformist lawyer who wanted, above all, to challenge American ideas about prurience and purity, was enlisted as an ally in the effort to publish texts that shared new information and attitudes toward sexuality. While written material that explained how individuals could avoid contracting disease or commented frankly on sexual longings broke new ground for American readers, old laws and moral codes persisted. Lingering concerns about decency and questions about copyright swirled in the background as the body of twentieth-century hygiene literature swelled, and this nexus was a choice ground for the views Schroeder wished to advance.

Hall and authors like him supplanted medically oriented works with sanitized, didactic treatises for the young, and, accordingly, scholarship has implied that conservative moral guidance substituted for what young people might have learned about sex during this period. Works which put forward sentimental and naive representations of sexuality and well-being formed only one portion of the market. Another was anchored by Fournier's explanations of how an individual could effectively fight syphilitic infection and Stall's encompassing account of the threats posed by gonorrhea, titles which provided rather specialized information to ordinary readers. Motivated, variously, by genuine interest in alleviating suffering and the potential rewards of publishing, authors committed scientific and medical details to print. The availability and the reception of the texts that carried such information, however, failed to echo the patterns of the first wave of science-based health texts for adolescents.

Sylvanus Stall, Theodore Schroeder, and the Saga of The Social Peril

Despite commercial success and repeated testimonials to the temperate nature of his texts, in 1905 Stall found himself the object of the least desirable attention a publisher could attract, as his competitors and

Anthony Comstock, leader of the New York Society for the Suppression of Vice, critically examined his enterprise. Stall advertised his Self and Sex Series in multiple venues, but he was engaged in other publishing opportunities as well. He printed any number of pamphlets, some designed to spur interest in his full-length works, and books including *The Social Peril,* which he promoted as a new title in the tradition of *What a Young Man Ought to Know.* In it, Stall addressed a "young man," speaking frankly and at length about venereal disease—focusing especially on gonorrhea—and other sexual problems, chiefly the failure to restrain one's sexual urges. He also celebrated the work of "United States postal authorities" in preventing the circulation of false and misleading health resources advertised in periodicals.[4]

On its face, the project was simply a parallel to Stall's other popular works; the objective was to make medical science that established the truly harmful nature of gonorrhea intelligible to ordinary readers. Stall explained that the book, which required his "prolonged preparation," "was largely written while crossing the ocean on a hurried business trip to and from London" with the aid of "a literary helper."[5] This minor narrative of the book's composition, Stall's accompanying statement of its urgent message, and his crediting "divine Providence" with its inspiration mattered little to two individuals. One was Dr. Prince A. Morrow, who accused Stall of plagiarizing his 1904 publication, *Social Diseases and Marriage.*[6] The other was Anthony Comstock. Their attention to this publication was responsible for generating its own series of interactions among prominent figures involved in the Progressive Era cause of providing sexual health information to adolescents. The fallout would be publicized later as an instance of Comstock's interference with even those who sought to encourage the morality that his vigilance was intended to ensure.[7]

The introduction to *Social Diseases and Marriage* might have been said to offer fair warning to imitators. Morrow proclaimed his work had the singular distinction of filling a tremendous void in the medical literature. He stated, "There is no comprehensive treatise in our language upon this subject, which has such important interests from both a medical and social point of view." Its innovation was this; earlier works, including Morrow's translation of Fournier's *Syphilis and Mar-riage,* had not emphasized the threat posed by gonorrhea. Then, Mor-row explained, it was still understood as a localized infection and one that women were inherently susceptible to; shortly after the turn of the century, this changed. "At the present day we recognize that the gono-coccus is the sole pathogenic agent in the immense majority of cases of a chronic or latent gonorrhea," Morrow wrote. In the course of this analysis, he would characterize "venereal diseases as a social peril."[8]

These factors aside, the two books have other features in common. Stall's practice of providing detailed tables of content for the books he published was continued in *The Social Peril,* and Morrow had employed the same technique in *Social Diseases and Marriage.* Morrow added a glossary at the end of his volume, while Stall provided footnotes to aid "the non-professional reader" with medical and scientific terms.[9] Still, Stall defined a number of words that Morrow did not, and Morrow's denotations retained the polysyllabic, technical vocabulary of medi-cine, while Stall endeavored to create understanding through a simpler wording.

In addition to these structural similarities, both authors were inclined to like means of addressing the fundamental problem of the spread of sexually transmitted infection. These views were ones both men had published before; moreover, complaints about the prolific transmission of syphilis and gonorrhea, demands for the education of the young, and, to borrow Morrow's words, concerns about "the degeneration of the race" were not unique to either. The two books conveyed related content, covering topics such as historical understandings of sexually transmitted infection and reversals of medical opinion about the treat-ment of gonorrhea, as well as the disease's effects on women and child-bearing. Morrow expressed concern about young men's ignorance and lust, ending his book with a call for the "persuasive force of enlighten-ment." He argued, in a blast of vehemence that Stall would have read-ily endorsed, "If a young man . . . is also instructed into a knowledge of the fact that venereal disease is the almost invariable concomitant of licentious living; that such indulgence is not wholesome for him; that it carries with it consequences to himself and others, often disastrous consequences, which may impair his health, vitiate his manhood, and lead to a forfeiture of all those hopes and aspirations which are to be fulfilled in a safe, fruitful, and happy marriage, he will pause and consider."[10] Stall's concluding call to the young man expressed similar sentiments, albeit with references to the importance of restraint and to "sexual endowment" as "a crowning gift of the Creator."[11] These resemblances were enough to lead Morrow to charge that Stall had plagiarized his work and violated his copyright.[12]

The wider world's first inklings of these events occurred in 1906. A letter from National Purity Federation president B. S. Steadwell brought news about the controversy surrounding Stall's book to the noted First Amendment attorney, Theodore Schroeder. Schroeder, a persistent and articulate gadfly who would gain further prominence during Emma Goldman's 1916 trial for disseminating birth control literature, had been engaged for some years in untangling legal and philosophical principles that he expected would demonstrate that "obscenity was nothing more than a subjective state of mind."[13] Schroeder was known for his allegiance to his own principles and helped to found the Free Speech League in 1902.[14] Among the individuals he aided were those who sought to avoid prosecution for publishing sexual health information, advising them about protective conventions they might invoke, like the doctor-patient relationship, and elements that would almost certainly lead to trouble, including explicitly stated facts and soliciting sales of one's work.[15]

Upon learning of the "suppression of the 'Vir' book," Schroeder sensed that the incident would yield a story congruent with his own interests.[16] He wrote to Stall, who replied shortly to acknowledge receipt of Schroeder's essay, "An Address on the Necessity for the Freedom of the Press in Relation to Sex," and to request a meeting.[17] Numerous conversations ensued, enabling Schroeder and Stall to become better acquainted. In spite of these men's prolonged contact, it was never a smooth relationship. Schroeder's interests, grounded in a complete rejection of conventional notions of indecency, were often at odds with Stall's religious convictions that brought him to a limited acceptance of the need to discuss human sexuality. Despite his initially sympathetic overtures, years later Schroeder would depict Stall as in the wrong in the conflict with Morrow over *The Social Peril*, stating that Stall had indeed "plagiarized a large part of the matter contained in a book by Dr. Prince A. Morrow."[18]

Schroeder identified Stall's reliance on an extensive passage describing the ruin of a young man who falls prey to the lure of a bordello as represented by Henry Ward Beecher, however, as the source of Comstock's complaint against the book.[19] He ascribed Comstock's attack on Stall as the outcome of Morrow's urging, mocking both prosecutor and victim, as well as revealing the dynamics behind alliances within the hygiene movement: "Not wishing to go to the expense of a law suit or gaining an injunction, he went to Anthony Comstock and asked him to suppress the Rev. Sylvanus Stall, D.D.'s book which contained the plagiarism. St. Anthony thought the material was obscene . . . [and] informed the Rev. SS DD that he must quit publishing of that book or be arrested and stand trial for obscenity. Dr. Stall suppressed the book."[20] For a man who livelihood was built on the foundation of decency, the threat of Comstock's public accusations was not an idle one. This title alone of the many produced by Vir Publishing is not mentioned in the periodical press or in the ads Stall included within each volume of the Self and Sex Series. Schroeder's anecdote indicates that even esteemed, long-standing partners within the Purity Movement were not immune to contemporary concerns about obscenity and that writers besides Stall were concerned with the market for their sexual health information treatises.

Stall and Schroeder would work together as part of the National Purity Federation's Committee on Obscenity Laws later that fall, and both, as well as Vir authors Mary Wood-Allen and Emma Drake, appeared on that year's program of the National Purity Conference.[21] The association wanted to modify obscenity laws used to harass individuals who disseminated hygiene literature, ostensibly at Schroeder's prompting, so the committee was charged with drafting a suitable resolution to present to the membership. Stall withheld his approval of the version Schroeder supported.[22] Schroeder nonetheless cooperated with other advocates for youthful purity. He published in the magazine of the National Purity Federation and spoke again at its annual conference.[23] Later, he would represent the group's concerns in Washington.[24]

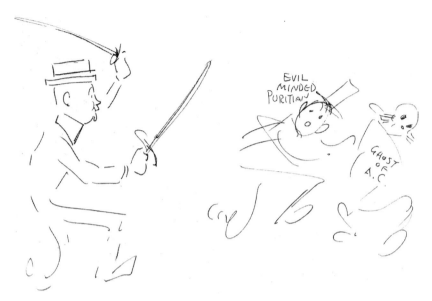

8. This sketch reveals a contemporary's perception of Theodore Schroeder as someone who fought valiantly against the puritanical hypocrisy promulgated by Anthony Comstock and those who shared his attitudes toward human sexuality. Special Collections Research Center, Morris Library, Southern Illinois University Carbondale. Reproduced with permission.

He corresponded with Rose Woodallen Chapman, editor of *American Motherhood* magazine and daughter of Vir Publishing's Mary Wood-Allen, who would reply "cordially" and in good humor to some of Schroeder's missives, although a falling out between the two eventually ensued.[25] He even attempted a correspondence with Comstock in 1906, seeking, he stated, to have Comstock reveal to him his errors in reasoning, but also requesting direct documentation of Comstock's censorship activities and goading the puritanical man with news of his own publications.[26] In the end, Schroeder seemed to have courted any number of tangled, temporary alliances with leaders of the hygiene movement for ambiguous reasons.

Though he was courteous to individuals during their lifetimes, when Schroeder recalled these interactions near the end of his own life he seemed to revel in his one-time associates' foibles. He intended to reveal potentially questionable aspects of these collaborators' lives, their clashes, and their failures to live according to the ideals they pro-

moted. Schroeder recalled Chapman was "handsome" but "quite flir-
tatious" and repeated a rumor that she had once traveled, unmarried,
to Europe with a man.[27] The daughter to whom *What a Young Woman
Ought to Know* was so "lovingly dedicated," he implied, had not pat-
terned her own life on the advice her mother urged upon others.[28]
Schroeder also condemned Morrow, to whose American Society for
Sanitary and Moral Prophylaxis he had once belonged, describing the
doctor's ground-breaking informational campaign as using "syphilis
as a scarecrow to induce people to lead continent lives."[29] He derided
Stall's interest as being less in securing protection from prosecution
than in having Comstock himself, who he alleged had shown him "his
choice and large collection" of books and photographs captured during
vice raids, arrested for "endangering his morals." After several meetings, Schroeder reported, "Of course I had to explain to him that I did
not believe in the objective reality of obscenity in any book, picture,
or play and therefore could give him no real assistance in the matter of
putting Mr. Comstock in jail."[30]

Read one way, Schroeder's recollections of Stall and the other Purity
Movement figures seem like petty, even spurious or malicious, gos-
sip. Another perspective on his recitation of conversations long past
is this: While these individuals marketed publications extolling their
passionately idealized representations of sexuality, their own lives,
under Schroeder's skeptical gaze, did not seem as innocent as they
proclaimed their young readers ought to be. Convictions that adolescents' conduct could be changed by hybrids of health information and
religious guidance did not mean that proponents found themselves
untroubled by sexual matters. Their published, commercial activity
differed, he seemed to suggest, from their private experiences. The
clash of these realities no doubt was intended to deflate, retrospec-
tively, the numinous interpretations of sex that filled the pages of the
Self and Sex Series. Most of the individuals about whom he wrote
were many years dead by the time he penned his accusing words, and
Schroeder never made his allegations public, failing to find funding
or a publisher for the account of his life that he drafted near its end.
And so that, as Schroeder ended so many chapters of his unpublished
autobiography, was the end of that story, offering only a brief, if tawdry

glimpse of the rivalries and the conflicts that threatened early twentieth-century hygiene publishing.

Winfield Scott Hall: The Clash of Science and Nostalgia

Stall's personal story of publishing success spun out at considerable
length. Before his empire came to an end, he found not just physicians
and vice prosecutors trying to unseat him as a pre-eminent publisher
of hygiene materials; other book people also contested his market position. Those who hoped to gain a share of his readers included the
Ladies' Home Journal editor Edward Bok, who once endorsed the Self
and Sex Series but went on to create his own line of hygiene titles, the
Edward Bok Books of Self-Knowledge for Young People and Parents.
These books were written, beginning in 1912, by writers well connected
to the American hygiene movement and the increasing number of
related for-profit publications. Among Bok's writers was Wood-Allen,
whom Stall had cultivated and Bok had once refused to print because
of concerns about the appropriateness of her work for the home reader;
as well as her daughter, Rose Woodallen Chapman, who worked with
the American Society for Sanitary and Moral Prophylaxis; and Winfield
Scott Hall, whose *Instead of Wild Oats: A Little Book for the Youth of
18 and Over* evoked Stall's American idiom and earlier French publications alike.[31] Wood-Allen's move to another publisher, even as Vir
continued to profit from her earlier manifestos, may have signified not
defection so much as her financial straits; however, Bok also had also
begun publishing the man who was perhaps Stall's strongest competitor, Winfield Scott Hall.

Hall, a doctor who used his credentials to argue for temperance
and other conservative causes, was among the writers who strove to
acquire the readership that Stall had galvanized with his recognizable
and acceptable texts. Hall's education and his extracurricular activities
anticipated the interests of his later career. On June 23, 1887, he became
part of what was then the largest graduating class at Northwestern University, one of thirty-four students to receive a baccalaureate diploma
that rainy morning. The commencement ceremony featured a speak-

ing contest, and an address on "The Conflict of the Races" signaled the developing interest Hall and his contemporaries had in eugenics.[32] This subject would form a continuing theme in Hall's professional activities as he gained expertise on the health and well-being of young people. Subsequently, in 1888, Northwestern recognized him with an award of $100 in prize money graduation for "the best all around examination in medicine, literature and science," the first of many distinctions he would win in the course of his career.[33]

Beginning with his years at Northwestern, groups like the YMCA claimed his attention and his intellectual leanings. As time passed and research produced new understandings of the teen years and the nature of venereal disease, Hall's popular writings bore the lingering marks of his avocation, rather than the advances of his profession. Still, not quite ten years after he joined the medical faculty of his alma mater, Hall was elected president of the American Academy of Medicine; at that time he was also president of the American Medical Temperance Association, a small, private group that required its members to pledge to abstain from alcohol and whose journal was published by Dr. John Harvey Kellogg.[34] This, together with other accolades, reflected Hall's increasing reputation, and likewise signaled his allegiances as he gained prominence in medical, educational, and reform communities.

Hall was both a member of Northwestern University's medical faculty and an ardent activist for Progressive Era reform interests, especially eugenics and race-related matters like the crusade against the so-called white slave trade that sought to eradicate both prostitution and sexual immorality.[35] He articulated his understanding of puberty in advice on diet and nutrition in his standard physiology text and a paper published by the Royal Anthropological Institute of Great Britain and Ireland that sought to define "the true American type."[36] Such works established Hall's expertise, demonstrated his embrace of eugenic principles, and made him a much-sought-after speaker and writer, particularly on social hygiene and adolescence. In turn, his interactions with advocacy groups that took up these causes led him from authoring mainstream physiology texts and articles in respected medical outlets to writing for organizations that wanted health treatises for young people.[37] His physician's credentials made his arguments compelling, a certain factor in the appeal of his texts. Yet Hall's popular treatises drew less on cutting-edge medical research than on moralistic assertions that impropriety—a staple reform concern in the first decades of the twentieth century—led directly to physical harm.

In addition to his own nostalgic ideals, Hall argued for chastity before and even within marriage. His, then, was a still more conservative voice urging readers to meet the threat of sexually transmitted infection with morality, arguing, at times, in others' words and on the basis of ever more dated medical findings. The backward glance at sexuality, in Hall's case, was not the result of nineteenth-century ministerial notions or an external perspective on the medical profession's efforts to treat those who suffered from syphilis. Hall affiliated with groups invested in ideas that had begun circulating during the previous century, before significant shifts had taken place in his profession's understanding of syphilis. In maintaining those connections, he advocated moral laws under the guise of modern medicine. Like Stall, though, Hall saw other activists embrace his conservative texts as ones that delivered important messages to young people and distribute them as part of their own groups' outreach efforts. Hall's hygiene texts depict another dimension of the intensely networked proliferation of sex education materials for adolescents during the Progressive Era; his profile as a physician, an author, and a one-time hygiene lecturer for the U.S. military indicates the advantages and the limitations that his position afforded him in his little acknowledged competition for the readership that Stall actively cultivated.

Whereas Stall concentrated his energies on a select number of publications, Hall approached writing differently. He was prolific, writing for the Young Men's Christian Association, the American Medical Association, and commercial publishers who formed the rapidly expanding industry that shared recent medical research with lay readers. In 1901, Hall published his first reproductive health instruction texts for children and their teachers.[38] Whether independently or with his wife and other co-authors, Hall went on to produce some fifty titles during his medical-writing career. This extensive catalogue, however, was not distinguished by originality and new ideas. While Hall's directives to young people became available through an increasing range of outlets, the information he produced had a static, sometimes even duplicative, quality. His many publications echoed one another, not infrequently reproducing content and structure from one volume to the next. *Sexual Knowledge: The Knowledge of the Self and Sex in Simple Language* and *From Youth into Manhood*, first printed in 1909 and reissued steadily until 1929 by the Young Men's Christian Association Press, were among his more popular works. During this time, the former title seemed poised to benefit from ads for Stall's well-known series, which were placed in magazines such as *McClure's* and *Life* using his long-standing "Self and Sex" phrase.[39] This reliance on another's work was far from an isolated episode in Hall's authorial endeavors.

Hall's stance on continence, or refraining from sexual activity except with the intent of conception, blended modern medical thinking with what one of his peers described elsewhere as medieval reasoning.[40] He acknowledged that intercourse was a pleasurable act for both men and women, yet his remarks on sexual health endorsed restraint, seeing sex as a procreative function that might be "indulged in . . . as often as once, twice per month."[41] Such moderation profited the young person, Hall wrote, in his grand yet vague notions of vigor and the inherent value of self-control. He therefore counseled young engaged couples who were planning their married lives to adopt separate beds, if not separate bedrooms, and in this was far more prescriptive than any work published by Stall.[42] While Hall was far from the only physician who encouraged this sort of restraint, others argued forcefully against it. Among them was William J. Robinson, editor of a handful of medical journals and *Sexual Truths,* a volume of essays by similarly avant-garde physicians who raised questions like "Is Platonic Love a Normal Relation?"[43] Demonstrably then, medical opinion on the relationship between sex and pleasure diverged rather sharply in these years. While Robinson did fierce battle with the views of Hall, the American Society for Sanitary and Moral Prophylaxis, and others who shared their conservative perspectives, Hall treated his opponent's ideas not as one man's thinking but as a general error to be denounced.[44]

Hall demonized gratuitous sexual activity, particularly masturbation. Although Havelock Ellis had trounced the specter of masturbatory harm as "ignorance and false tradition" in 1900, Hall adamantly adhered to, and published, older scientific conclusions.[45] He authoritatively told young women who might be tempted to regard auto-erotic impulses as harmless that masturbation "is universally recognized as an abuse of the organs and a diversion of their function from the normal." The consequences of this "serious shock to her nervous system" included its wreckage, he warned.[46] In advising parents of the importance of deterring a teen's developing sexual urges through attitudes fostered in childhood, Hall deliberated the common belief in a link between masturbation and insanity. Although an increasing number of prominent experts followed Ellis in debunking the connection, Hall maintained, "Even if it should be demonstrated as true that self-abuse may cause insanity, much the strongest motive for right living is to be found in painting .the glories, wonders, and beauties of the ideal and perfect manhood and womanhood, and simply warning the child that indulgence in the wrong habit will mar this beauty and perfection, and cause him to fall short of the ideal."[47] Decades into the twentieth century then, Hall's views resonated with what D'Emilio and Freedman have called "the shrill pronouncements of some nineteenth-century writers that youthful masturbation led to insanity."[48] Through his efforts, strictures against self-gratification became ensconced as a distinctive part of the American for-profit hygiene treatise for adolescents.

His program of pure thoughts and chaste actions, he declared, would prevent disease and prepare young people to become satisfied marital partners and parents, seldom acknowledging the changing and challenging research that was shared at conferences, in medical journals, and via the circulation of manuscripts in the professional com-munity. Instead, he articulated views derived from contemporary thinking about adolescence, especially by activists convinced that sex education staved off potential crises and ruin. *Girlhood and Its Problems: The Sex Life of Woman* was written with his wife to provide "a guide for girls, young women, young wives and young mothers; answering their questions and giving instruction which should guide the young woman into healthy, happy, wifehood and proud, efficient motherhood" because, as he continued, "Every normal young woman wishes to be a home builder, —a wife and mother."[49] These beliefs, though shared by many in the medical profession, were a secondary stream of thinking that did not replace ongoing efforts to cure and even to prevent diseases such as syphilis.

In the companion volume, *Youth and Its Problems: The Sex Life of a Man,* Hall contended that acting in accord with honorable and patriotic sentiments saved U.S. forces from venereal disease during World War I.[50] While Hall attributed the health of military men to the guidance that he put forth, government reports presented a somewhat different story.[51] Hall failed to inform readers of this volume about the availability of Salvarsan or other contemporary remedies; the Navy's Surgeon General, however, documented the medical treatment of venereal disease and highlighted new prevention measures, chiefly the detainment of suspected prostitutes, that made it "possible to attack the problem openly in the civil community."[52] David Pivar has described the military's emphasis on personal purity in this era, an emphasis that Hall helped create, but it is evident that the Navy implemented education, medication, and legal measures to reduce infection.[53] It was a nonetheless imperfect plan. Despite his initially confident assertions, one year later a report by the Navy's Surgeon General would show that rates of syphilis and gonorrhea had spiked again.[54] Hall's claims for his work, then, attempted to capitalize on a blend of optimism and postwar patriotism, rather than the actualities of military medical practice, and in doing so kept the focus on adolescents' personal conduct rather than widening his scope to include information on treatment for a reader who had ever strayed from the chaste ideals he proffered. Such cautious clinging to the medical past, however, ascertained that the sale of his works would go unchallenged.

Both of Hall's companion books, though their titles promised to clarify a young person's ideas about reproduction and relations between the sexes, merely enjoined readers to avoid smoking, drinking, or engaging in sexual activity with anything other than procreative motives. He use jargon spawned by advocates of social hygiene and sex education to discuss adolescents' "life problems" or sexual conduct. The domestic goals of marriage and raising a family, a norm endorsed by nearly every writer of hygiene treatises, could be achieved only if teenagers governed their sexual impulses, they reasoned. Anything that might encourage licentiousness was to be discouraged. Although Columbia University professor Maurice Bigelow challenged prevailing ideas about adolescence, he agreed with those who saw a young person's sexuality as essentially fraught, writing that "the hygienic and educational problems of adolescence are often popularly and correctly referred to as 'the problems of the teens.'"[55] Hall, in 1913, put the matter plainly: "The physical well-being of the adolescent and of the adult depends very largely upon a healthy condition of the sex organs, and his moral well-being upon a right mental attitude toward sex subjects."[56] Thus human sexuality remained linked to general health when the ability to cure syphilis was still new, imperfect, and disputed; that reproduction warranted direction on moral living echoed a much longer tradition which publishers adapted to present-day concerns. Hall's works suggested that the certainties of sexual continence were safer than the evolving steps toward effective treatment and that adolescents should not be trusted with knowledge that might encourage them to make choices other than the ones he deemed correct.

His ideological leanings in these youth-oriented titles were more than simply conservative, and his characteristic medical nostalgia became more pronounced over time as Hall emphatically promoted social laws said to mirror natural ones that a number of physicians and experts on adolescence had begun to reject. While his books featured cut-section diagrams of reproductive organs and referenced the theories of prominent researchers, scientific aspects of his publications competed with eugenic views intended to secure, as contemporary reformers expressed it, the future of the race. Yet his prolific publications indicate that his agenda found adherents among professionals and reformers, and among publishers and the readers who purchased their titles.

Collectively, this body of work led eugenicist Paul Popenoe to describe Hall, in 1927, as someone who had been "for nearly a generation," "one of the most active writers and lecturers in the field of social hygiene."[57] Even following his retirement from Northwestern's medical school in 1919, Hall's perspective on adolescent health and well-being was still sought. He became affiliated with the International University in Brussels, a "project . . . endorsed by the Council of the League of Nations" that was intended to bring together the "ablest professors" and the "elite of the world's students."[58] Hall was also president of the Child Conservation League, whose board included the psychologist G. Stanley Hall and several prominent eugenicists.[59]

He contributed to books like *The Child: His Nature and His Needs.*[60] This volume, first published by the Children's Foundation in 1924 and reprinted multiple times throughout the decade, offered teachers, social workers, and parents a survey of current research by noted physicians and faculty at leading American institutions.[61] Hall's chapter on adolescence reflected the credibility he had established during his career as a physician and author, which emerged in tandem with the child-study movement and the subsequent attention that psychologists, scientists, and physicians directed to the transition between childhood and adult life.[62] As Popenoe rather belatedly noted though, Hall's advice contained "numerous errors of fact or emphasis" that detracted from its "high ideals."[63] It was not a judgment that carried much weight during Hall's lifetime.

Hall's works were undeniably popular, and professionals who used his treatises to support their work with teens reported that wide distribution of his writings provoked no protests. This was particularly true of a series of four pamphlets published under the auspices of the AMA in 1913.[64] These short narratives, which sold for a quarter apiece, explained elements of reproduction as the title characters conversed with their parents about the vagaries of female maturation and the wonders of life's beginnings as witnessed at an uncle's farm. One of the AMA booklets, "John's Vacation: What John Saw in the Country," bore more than a passing resemblance to a translation of a Swedish pamphlet, "How My Uncle the Doctor Instructed Me in Matters of Sex," produced by the American Society for Sanitary and Moral Prophylaxis almost a decade before.[65] The Swedish translation was simultaneously in print, being promoted as a resource in 1911.[66] This short work affords the clearest and most direct evidence that Hall looked to the ideas and texts that other authors made popular, taking cues, concepts, and sometimes even the words themselves from treatises already in circulation.

Despite their stilted tone and their relatively late introduction, Hall's

AMA titles demonstrated a not inconsiderable appeal. Three years or more after their initial publication, the booklets, which modeled parent-child instruction, emphasized premarital abstinence, and articulated social laws governing morality, remained in print. In Maine, a private committee of physicians gave out thousands of copies of Hall's stories featuring John's earnest if didactic dialogues with his father, and the group reported with satisfaction that they received no complaints, despite having solicited them. F. N. Whittier, head of the state's Committee on Venereal Diseases and Their Prevention, attributed the success of Hall's work to the shifting sentiments of the American public: "Parents are beginning to realize the necessity of early instruction in matters of sex. The social diseases, a few years ago a forbidden discussion, are receiving the consideration of many thoughtful citizens. The public believes more than ever before that modern hygienic methods should be applied to all communicable diseases."[67] The public's notion of modernity, however, was misplaced. Even years before the publication of the AMA series, Hall's pronouncements no longer represented the vanguard of medical thought. For all the complaints that it had, by 1906, become "Sex O' Clock in America," by 1916, and for many years thereafter, the wide audiences for Hall's treatises for young people reflected belief in another time altogether. The staid health advice put forward by Hall belied a simple truth: these years saw nearly continuous advances in the understanding of human reproduction and the treatment of sexually transmitted infection. This shifting terrain created disparities in information disseminated to the public, too, as some physicians and reformers sought to differentiate valid conclusions from less credible material, while others employed the inevitable ambiguities in research findings to shore up personal, moralistic attitudes toward sexuality.

Hall, during his lifetime, contended for the readership that Stall had cultivated, although the scientific and medical research that fostered Hall's rise as an expert on adolescence was eclipsed in these popular writings by the ideologies that shaped his personal beliefs. Hall's writings for adolescent readers selectively invoked the new science while positioning his value-driven perspective as the logical unfolding of medical research. Although there were books that expressed decidedly more liberal attitudes toward sex, Stall's primary competitor was, if anything, more conservative. Morality was less challenging than medical facts, and Hall's messages suited the market.

The Further Work of Alfred Fournier

Regardless of the apparent conservatism of the American book market, Fournier had made inroads into this territory during the course of his career. English-language translations and reviews of his study of syphilis were no rarity in the nineteenth century. Although Morrow has been credited with translation of the French doctor's lengthy treatise, *Syphilis and Marriage,* he was neither the first nor the last to make the French syphilographer's research available to American readers. In England, the New Sydenham Society had regularly incorporated Fournier's work into the annual volumes it sold to English and American subscribers.[68]

Short papers about his clinical activities also abounded in U.S. medical periodicals all through the final decades of the nineteenth century. Particularly when Fournier offered a contention about syphilis that nettled American dignity, as when he reopened the question of whether the disease was brought back to Europe from the new world, American physicians seemed ready to engage him.[69] U.S. medical publications offered every sort of awareness of the Frenchman's medical opinions: reviews of his books, translations of individual lectures, and reports of how his thinking conflicted with or supported another physician's ideas about syphilis made Fournier the leading expert on syphilis not just in Paris, but in America as well, even before English-language editions of his works appeared.[70] Thus, Morrow's preface to his own translation that insisted "there is not, that I am aware, any work in the English language which treats of the relations of syphilis with marriage" was somewhat overstated.[71] The subject of *Syphilis and Marriage* was a long-established area of investigation for Fournier and one that had already been introduced to American medical practitioners.[72]

In addition to the more technical material he wrote for his fellow practitioners, Fournier offered readers accessible renditions of medical information that acknowledged both the potential to cure syphilis and the general public's ability to understand the technicalities of treatment. The significance of his publications advising ordinary individuals that a return to health was indeed possible cannot be overstated, either in contemporary or historical context. Fournier's colleagues, in their memorials of the distinguished physician, credited him with two slim volumes for readers outside the medical community; published early in the twentieth century; *En guérit-on?* and *Pour en guérir* repeated the themes of *Pour nos fils* but also analyzed, in some detail, the best extant treatments for syphilis.[73]

Adolescents who could follow the vocabulary and the reasoning presented in the "For Our Children" treatises would have had no difficulties with Fournier's later popular works, which depended on a plain style and, chemical references aside, a simple approach to medical care. The most effective chemical compounds and the optimal duration of treatment were revealed clearly and openly in *En guérit-on?*, his 1906 book, and its more emphatic revision a year later. In these titles, intended to support syphilitic patients' recovery, Fournier explained the state of medicine so that the reader might select a good doctor and abide by the prescribed regimen, regardless of the unpleasantness of the course. This explanation to ordinary readers, regardless of age, was published decades after his translated research conclusions had begun circulating among British and American doctors.[74] When these new volumes that expressed the conviction that a return to health was possible and the means of ensuring it made their way to America, however, it was in the original French, as he reserved his rights to these texts.

In *En guérit-on?* and *Pour en guérir,* however, Fournier crafted documents unlike any others on the market. These treatises assured the stricken, "Yes, we can fight it. Yes, under certain conditions that I will tell you, we can fight syphilis."[75] By blending encouragements, caveats, and treatment regimens, Fournier once again committed to print what few others dared. His advocacy of long-term courses of mercury and potassium iodate, which he called "the two therapeutic pearls," was elaborated over some one hundred pages.[76] Although Fournier did not fail to repeat his by then standard warnings about protecting the health of family and nation, he offered counsel on all aspects of life that might affect the patient's recovery. Alcohol was among these topics, singled out for its tendency to worsen the skin conditions associated with syphilis and the way syphilis affected the nervous system, which he saw as contributing to paralysis.[77] The duration of treatment, based on different presentations of the disease, was outlined in these works through case histories. Regardless of how long individuals had been afflicted, once therapy was established, they gained relief, Fournier promised. Lest sufferers fear they could not afford medical care, Fournier noted that because evidence indicated ailing individuals initially ineligible for state aid only worsened while waiting for care, rules that made a period of residency a condition of free treatment had been suspended.[78]

Fournier acknowledged the worst-case scenarios, yet believed, in the end, that patients required more than medical care; they were also entitled, he argued, to hope. He envisioned an invalid who followed the advice in *En guérit-on?* saying to himself, "It's a battle between the malady and me. To work, then, and courage! Courage, since science affirms that with mercury, hygiene, and time, we can come to the end of syphilis, and since science gives me hope of one day recovering my health and besides, of having the right to aspire to have a family, with the liberty and the happiness to become a father!"[79] Much as he had imagined himself in conversation with those who could benefit from his knowledge when he initiated science-based publications for the common reader, Fournier again saw himself speaking, with goodwill and a professional lifetime's knowledge, to those in need.

Evidence arising from the later work of Fournier, Stall, and Hall indicates that authors' motives for their public communications about venereal disease were decidedly yet sometimes legitimately mixed, involving profit and proprietary rights as well as public health. For someone like Fournier, such self-protection was warranted both by French legal tradition and by the fact that others published his research to augment their professional reputations and incomes.[80] The refusal of the United States government to authorize the Berne Convention that guarded intellectual property in Europe made efforts to control the international dissemination of a text that much more difficult. Thus, an important work like *Pour en guérir* was far more limited in its American impact, although physicians discussed its promise.[81]

Developments surrounding the publications by these three men showed that controlling the way one's ideas were represented in print mattered. When an individual in one country might, effectively, claim proceeds from a medical or scientific work created by considerable labor elsewhere, reserving the rights to that material was a logical outgrowth of unauthorized reproductions, especially given the new and increasing market for sexual health material in the early twentieth century. Without the ability to rely on Fournier's leadership in syphilis research and public education, it seems, too, that technicality of commercial English-language texts for nonprofessional audiences began to fall into abeyance. Later publications made available by nonprofit organizations, though seldom reaching the circulation figures of earlier titles, nonetheless made an effort to share something of the more familiar facts behind disease. One, a 1916 treatise promoted by a New York health agency, sounded familiar themes for adolescent readers. Like the first French pamphlets and Hurty's treatise, it rehearsed the means of contracting syphilis, listing "kissing, swapping pipes, by common use of such utensils as glasses, drinking cups, towels, etc." In a way reminiscent of Fournier's first work, the writer asked would-be fathers, after a description of the consequences of syphilitic infection, "Can you willfully leave such a legacy to your future children?"[82] For some time, appeals for adolescent chastity went untouched by scientific developments.

Much recent scholarship on the historic development of prevention treatises has implied that authors intended the moral tenor of these works to substitute for medical advances. Yet for years after the patenting of Salvarsan and prior to the discovery of penicillin, a stream of white papers and research reports on treatment circulated internationally. Physicians thus pursued the most effective means of easing infected patients' conditions, and the pharmaceutical industry advertised wares to aid treatment in professional publications.[83] The circulation of typescript translations of documents like "An Exact Serology Guides the Treatment of Syphilis" meant doctors in the United States could avail themselves of any advances that took place abroad, regardless of language barrier.[84] The effects of venereal disease on even the very young were considered in these medical works: "The advantages of the simultaneous, combined salvarsan-mercury treatment include this one, that a correct application of the method removes all possibility of pain. . . . Therefore the treatment is especially suited for syphilitic infants, in whom the cranial and brachial veins still protrude too slightly to admit of a puncture."[85] To suggest, as some scholarly literature has, that physicians relied on morality as a substitute for treatment, goes too far.

Implicit in scholarly critiques of older treatises on sex and disease is the notion that such texts were more conservative than they ought to have been. The publishing history of Fournier, Stall, and Hall, though, suggests that several factors effectively demanded that writers at least nod to traditional values by treating the subject of sex with circumspection. The encounter between Stall and Comstock, spurred by a physician's claims of infringement, indicates that the content of health texts for young people could provoke prosecution. Further, if practitioners with the increasingly technical knowledge involved in treating disease claimed that what they knew was proprietary, it became more difficult for publishers like Stall to distribute more scientific information. Controversy in France over the appropriateness of the French Society's pamphlets, and the iterations of the efforts to make sharing reproductive health information acceptable, particularly with young women, likewise reflected cultural resistance to more radical proclamations; certainly, those who followed the doings of the French Society were aware that more liberal information efforts netted controversy rather than adherence. The commercial appeal of works like those produced by Hall also suggested that conservative tracts, rather than avant-garde or frank ones, had the strongest commercial appeal in the United States.

Further, Comstock's apparent willingness to prosecute medical information as unsavory material must have prompted caution. Not long after the investigation that Schroeder documented, the American Medical Association warned its members that the prosecution of the mailing of indecent materials could be extended to clinical and research treatises that were standard professional reading matter.[86] While Comstock sought to limit the circulation of any potentially indelicate material, his foremost goal was protecting the young.[87]

The title of his self-justifying treatise, *Frauds Exposed; Or How the People are Deceived and Robbed, and Youth Are Corrupted*, pointed to the problem Comstock saw himself addressing by censorship: "My object is to . . . shield our youth from debauching and corrupting influences; to arouse a public sentiment against the vampires who are casting deadly poison into the fountain of moral purity in the children."[88] He continued his diatribe against writers and publishers whose work might harm children, citing the example of physicians who used their knowledge of the body, he claimed, to produce "obscene literature [that] . . . secretly eats out the moral life and purity of our youth, and they droop and fade before their parents' eyes."[89] Like the men who drafted hygiene treatises, Comstock, too, avowed that he strove to protect young people. Unlike many influential hygiene authors, however, he saw "devil-traps for the young" where others saw providing information about sex and the body as a critical means of ensuring adolescents would not be trapped by ill health or lengthy, painful medical treatment.[90] The vice-inspector's pervasive influence, which he described in terms of a few plays closed, hundreds of people arrested for purveying indecent material, tens of thousands of pounds of texts and printing equipment seized, and miles traveled in pursuit of malefactors, created inherent risks for individuals who produced scientifically oriented hygiene texts.[91]

Hygiene writers' reservations about the uses to which their texts and ideas might be put, however, did not mean these individuals lacked compassion or sensitivity to the plight of the infected. American commentaries on *En guérit-on?* noted the appropriateness of its message, and long before, when the Sydenham Society translated Fournier's research for English-speaking doctors, they also published a parallel essay on treating syphilis. Its author noted that controversy over the effects and the duration of mercury prevailed among the medical community, with implications that were little considered:

> This subject has recently been under discussion by German dermatologists, and Fournier's method of intermittent treatment of prolonged

duration was strenuously advocated by me in opposition to the older method of expectant and symptomatic treatment upheld by Caspari, Pick, Jarisch, Kaposi, Gluck, Havas, Petersen, Mracek, and others. The general consensus of opinion opposed Fournier's method, which a small minority supported. . . . It is not a question, however, of majorities, whether one or the other side wins, but one of humanity, on which it is most important to arrive at as correct a decision as possible.[92]

The many and complex perspectives that arose from the ways that venereal disease was regarded around the world were seldom negotiated without considering humanity, and all its strengths and weaknesses. The exponential difficulties in publishing sexual health information treatises early in the twentieth century sometimes meant efforts to minimize young people's chances of being afflicted by either serious illness or protracted treatments faded and became distant concerns. In an anxious world, writers and publishers found they had to safeguard themselves and their work against opportunists and zealots, rather than concentrating solely on whatever protections their words might afford adolescents.

CONCLUSION

*I have to thank you for forwarding to us the six issues of 'Social
Diseases,' which will make a complete set with the number that we
have. The Library's funds for its subscriptions to periodicals are out of
proportion to the demands made upon them, for which reasons gifts
from publishers of their publications are most welcome. Should you see
your way clear . . . to placing the Library's name on your mailing list,
we would be glad to make it available to all proper inquirers.*

—JOHN SHAW BILLINGS, DIRECTOR OF THE
NEW YORK PUBLIC LIBRARY, TO THE
AMERICAN SOCIAL HYGIENE ASSOCIATION

Their difficult inception a recent but fading memory, the initial sexual
and reproductive health titles of the twentieth century were soon awash
in competition. Where Alfred Fournier had once envisioned himself
alone, counseling a father to share *Pour nos fils* with his adolescent
sons, there followed any number of publishers who wished to join this
conversation and thrust their works into a bewildered parent's hands.
A mere five years after the imaginary and then seemingly idealistic col-
loquy, the outpourings of writers determined to publish their thoughts
about sex for younger readers had reached unanticipated proportions.
Much as the sudden surfeit of sexual health texts then prompted recon-
sideration of what adolescents ought to know, the networks of print
that produced these works now invite scholarly reassessment of the
theories that have explained earlier scientific and print culture.

That transatlantic connections eventually made authoring hygiene
titles almost ordinary, rather than revolutionary, is evident. The veritable flood of information created new dilemmas for those involved in its
production and distribution, whether authors or government officials,
and especially well-intentioned parents. When should they broach the
subject of reproduction? How should they instruct their children in

hopes of avoiding the dire problems of which experts warned? In time, these questions became a single one: which book suited their child? As his agenda succeeded, Fournier's guidance, not just for young men but for the guardians who chose texts on sex and reproduction for the young readers in their care, seemed almost as necessary as the technical facts he provided. Renewed attention to reading guidance, as well as reading material, emerged from efforts to convey disease prevention messages to new audiences. Adults who confronted the inadequacies of their own knowledge wanted information to guide their decisions, as well as works that their children might safely read.[1]

Recommenders typically met the challenge of choosing such books for young people with confidence, and venturing opinions about appropriate titles soon became a convention of hygiene tracts. Sometimes, as in the works issued by Vir Publishing, the suggestions for further reading were self-referential and explicitly promotional, publicizing "valuable books" sold by the press.[2] Elsewhere, the aim seemed mild and expansive, seeing the reading of "books of instruction and of wholesome adventure" as sufficient to the aim of discouraging dangerous youth-ul vice.[3] Particularly as the genre matured, publishers positioned themselves as part of a respectable community, possessing suitable knowledge and values, through their endorsements. Seldom, however, did these referrals reflect the intense personal communication and the extensive dispersal of texts that had begun in 1901.

Regardless of the broader effects wrought by these powerful connections, some hesitation remained. The American Library Association, in responding to librarians' questions about reproductive health materials suitable for their collections, appeared to defer to the judgment of the American Social Health Association. Yet of nearly two-dozen titles deemed useful by the hygiene collective, librarians learned that only a few should be considered essential purchases.[4] This modest counsel was one of a mere four articles on hygiene literature in libraries published during these years of scientific change and reform campaigns.[5] Nor did the professional literature mention that the ASHA offered libraries a traveling collection of key titles that could be borrowed for only the cost of postage, although the New York Public Library acknowledged the importance of the association's donation of materials in light of budget shortfalls.[6] State associations also emulated this strategy of trying to place volumes in libraries.[7] The relative silence of the professional library literature suggests one reason that, in 1912, ASHA officers planned marketing campaigns directly to libraries.[8] Although others believed in their potential to provide the public with sexual health information, librarians were reserved. They were not alone in their cautious treatment of sexual health texts.

Other experts clearly articulated their doubts about the increasingly sought-after commodity of hygiene literature. The psychologist G. Stanley Hall accumulated "a large bookcase full of literature on this subject" only to judge nearly all of it wanting. He scoffed that a "ten-minute talk" would serve better than any book in his possession.[9] When an expert like Hall promoted old-fashioned conversation over recently printed works, individuals whose livelihood depended on the written word worried whether his statements might deflate the market they had cultivated. Accordingly, publishers reinforced their efforts to make print integral to parental responsibilities with promises of pure thinking and problem-solving. In advice on child-raising, parents' needs were met with hygiene publishers' commercial messages.

Ladies' Home Journal, for example, enhanced its marketing and responded to the concerns of uncertain but earnest parents by introducing the column "How Shall I Tell My Child?"[10] Written by Rose Woodallen Chapman, daughter of Sylvanus Stall's leading author and herself a speaker for the American Society for Sanitary and Moral Prophylaxis, the monthly commentary counseled mothers about how to provide age-appropriate information while protecting youthful innocence. Her voice countered Hall's, her feminine tone and sensibilities delicately, if indirectly, indicating reasons that readers should purchase the titles she and her mother wrote. Such strategies enhanced the broad appeal of books and maintained the centrality of early purveyors.

The economics of publishing aside, in promoting health through reading, reformers influenced the concept of adolescence as a cultural phenomenon, the acceptance of advances in science and medicine, and the ways these ideas made their way into print. It follows, then, that scholarly reflection on the authorial activities of Fournier and those who emulated his work responds in turn to theories that account for historic scientific and print cultures. Two landmark theoretical constructs underscore an analysis of the profusion of science-based sexual health texts for young readers. The first is Thomas Kuhn's theory of scientific revolutions, which has modeled the means by which new scientific ideas become the norm, and the second is Robert Darnton's communications circuit, which has defined and shaped print culture studies.[11] Early twentieth-century hygiene literature, crafted by networks of scientists and publishers alike, presents a case for augmenting these explanatory frameworks in light of the attention writers and activists directed to young people's reading.

Reading Progressive Era sexual health literature for adolescents and reconstructing its dynamic, even turbulent contexts involves real, and provocative individuals and texts. The human feelings that gave rise to attempts to meet young people's need to understand their changing bodies and sex are striking, even when captured in a colleague's remembrances or the perspectives conveyed in more technical documents; together they reveal the strong convictions, personal frailties and foibles, and high, if sometimes blind, ideals behind these projects. If evidence of proponents' shortcomings remains, the strength of their convictions and their sustained commitment to the ordinary adolescent, who they expected would mature into a mother or father, were pronounced and consequential.

Kuhn posits that scientific revolution occurs when one explanation contends with an extant view and the former displaces the older, irreconcilable account of a scientific phenomenon.[12] Before the end of the nineteenth century Fournier aspired to this sort of foundational change, attributing venereal disease to microbes rather than to people or place and insisting that these ailments represented serious and, for a time, irremediable harm. Even though his work fell outside the domain of what Kuhn called "normal science" or, to employ a more recent idiom, the hard sciences, the starting point for Fournier's public health campaign was the clinical demonstration of the severity and the unmitigated contagiousness of syphilitic infection. His aim of changing medical approaches to treatment and prevention approximates Kuhn's criterion that a revolutionary paradigm shift alters "the scientific imagination in ways that we shall ultimately need to describe as a transformation of the world in which scientific work was done."[13] Fournier indeed asked his colleagues to reconceive the province of medicine, a legacy his students and prominent physicians later honored.

What distinguishes Fournier's writings from the ones that Kuhn postulated as revolutionary is the human element intrinsic to medical practice. Fournier investigated diseases that grievously afflicted individuals, whose illness constituted the "external social need" that Kuhn acknowledged as an aspect of medicine in his account of scientific research.[14] Fournier wrote in the midst of an as yet unsettled scientific era, when despite earlier scientific discoveries, germ theory failed to serve as an explanatory force for the transmission of venereal disease. Other doctors' persistent doubt makes clear that professional opinion had yet to coalesce around bacteria as the cause of venereal disease. Into this gap researchers and clinicians poured theories that had flourished for decades. The end Fournier sought, however, was to see that improved scientific understanding of disease fundamentally changed medical, governmental, and social responses to individuals and their illnesses.

This ambition directs researchers who endeavor to understand that process and the texts it produced to seek evidence of new paradigms beyond the scientific community, in popular culture and realms where scientists spoke not to each other but to the public. When the effects of scientific change are profound, they will be observed outside the laboratory and the specialized discourse of the research community, informing the way people understand their lives and what they teach their children. In initiating this sexual health campaign and authoring its first popular text, Fournier sought nothing less.

Chief among those whom Fournier thought and wrote about were young people. His writings and the parallel works of his colleagues identified adolescence as a time when both reproductive capability and sexual feelings developed, when the young person left home and became more independent. While his conflation of puberty and adolescence might not withstand scrutiny informed by twenty-first century research, it was nonetheless influential among his contemporaries.

Describing young people in these terms was innovative and made the ideas expressed in *Pour nos fils* and *Pour nos filles*, central to the concerns of American reformers in the coming years.

In all these publications, adolescence was a prolonged condition. It began with the teen years, and it extended into one's twenties. This protracted stage of life, rather than infantilizing the maturing young person, anticipates recent reconceptualizations of adolescence stemming from the neurological research of Jay Giedd and Ronald Dahl.[15] Thus, given concerns about the strength and influence of family relations, most early twentieth-century writers used terms like *child* or *children* even when they referred to young adults. As understood by a number of recent scholars, the cultural phenomenon of adolescence developed from an increase in leisure and a relative surfeit of useful labor, tandem conditions which made it desirable and even necessary to extend the years before a young person entered the work force.

Considered from the perspective of contemporary reformers, however, it was young people's entry into the urban work force that created many of the difficulties associated with adolescence. As historian Jeffrey Moran has observed, "With the transportation revolution that began around 1815, young men were increasingly abandoning agriculture for commercial and industrial occupations. They fled not only their parents' traditional occupations but also the adult community's supervision and protection."[16] Moran overstates, however, cultural restrictions on young women (and thus undercounts hygiene treatises intended for a female readership) who likewise left rural homes for jobs in the city, a situation to which reformers attributed many a moral failing. Jane Addams was prominent among those who decried the living conditions of young women employed in New York's factories, citing "the possibilities of secrecy in a big city" as a reason "why girls go wrong."[17] Her endorsement of a "protective league organized among working girls to enable the big army of girls in the industrial field to help each other," a collective which made thousands of visits in its efforts to care for hundreds and hundreds of young women, signals their considerable presence in American cities by the first decade of the twentieth century.[18] Addams saw men as cads and criminals, and young women as their hapless victims, a point of view that extended from individuals to the gendered texts that warned them against the ruin of their morals and their health.

Of the plentiful, prescriptive texts for male and female readers, a small number were particularly important as reflected by print-runs, translations, imitations, outright duplications, and recommendations that young people read them. The individuals who produced these more significant texts knew, or at least knew of, one another. Their relationships fostered discussion and reflection upon their mutual endeavors; consequently, it is possible to uncover the nature of hygiene authorship and publication. Tracing the communications that forged relationships among authors, publishers, and distributors reveals the different ways in which influential treatises gained international audiences. Analyzing these connections enables us to see, as Darnton has written, "how ideas were transmitted through print and how exposure to the printed word affected the thought and behavior of mankind."[19]

Dialogue surrounding the dissemination of early twentieth-century hygiene treatises for young readers indicates that tensions were inherent in the process of putting still developing, controversial ideas into print, however noble the rationale. It is clear that no single mechanism facilitated the publication of health-oriented work for young people in the first decades of the twentieth century; cumulatively, however, reproductive health texts were widely distributed and effectively shifted the means of sex education from conversation to print. Their influence was nonetheless simply the first of many successive waves of efforts to see that young lives would not be cut short by uninformed choices. Then as now, social and legal contexts dissuaded the production of health treatises, while medical and commercial forces fostered it.

There are, in these early texts, apparent anticipations of more recent preoccupations in textual creation and distribution. Skepticism about its actual merits notwithstanding, twenty-first-century writers discuss the long-tail economics of self-publishing and small-scale distribution to individual readers rather than stores. A publisher like Sylvanus Stall, who produced a limited number of titles and reached out to buyers through one-to-one merchandising and specialized outlets, had already realized the potential of marketing to individuals, rather than depending on continuous store presence or mass-media advertisements. Meetings where pamphlets were available, letters from distant petitioners, or the good opinion of a neighbor or a colleague who passed on a particular hygiene title represented other typical means of acquiring early health information texts. The technologies that today reduce the effort and the time required for global communication did not exist when Fournier, Stall, and others who published early hygiene treatises strove to convey health information to adolescents, yet they clearly anticipated the models, if not the modes, of modern communication and commerce. Early twentieth-century reliance on small presses, personal marketing, and dispersed sales outlets that appear, when considered in broad terms, as precursors to more contemporary marketing strategies, suggests some discrepancies between actual historic operations and enduring ideas about how books come to be read.

The communications circuit that frames scholarly discussion of print culture was conceived, initially, as a mechanism that accounted for the book-selling practices of eighteenth-century France. Its broader utility is undeniable, and yet, documents that remain to reveal the material and cultural conditions of other places and times indicate that writers and publishers, at times, did not rely on others to refine, print, and distribute their works. In the case of early twentieth-century hygiene treatises, for instance, the roles of author, editor, publisher, and promoter were all performed by the small entities and individuals who developed health texts for adolescent readers. Translations that made health messages accessible in multiple nations were a factor in creating readership, yet they were not always controlled or approved by the authors of the original texts. Distribution was likewise either one more element of a concentrated and centralized process or, in contrast, decentralized and dependent on secondary publishers, door-to-door salespeople, or readers who passed along personal copies. These variances had to do with whether producers prioritized disease prevention messages or the potential for profit, as well as their related institutional context. The specialized and typically small information producers of the early twentieth century are not well explained with reference to a circuit, despite the communicative intent motivating their formation.

Still, as Paul Erickson has observed, Darnton's model raises "many of the right questions when trying to understand the explosion of print" in other contexts.[20] Notably, early twentieth-century hygiene literature calls for greater emphasis on elements that Darnton characterizes as background rather than foreground. Given the general controversy and the specific legal issues historically involved in publishing sexual health information, abstractions such as "intellectual influences and publicity," "economic and social conjecture," and "political and legal sanctions" are crucial considerations.[21] These contextual factors influenced everything from a hygiene publication's title and the way it was advertised to its very existence.

Further, multiple contexts and paratextual elements demonstrate the strong connections among authors of sexual health treatises for adolescents. Darnton notes that authors are readers, even though he simultaneously deemphasizes that link with a dotted line in visual depictions of his communications circuit. It is evident, though, that the authors of hygiene titles read each other's work and corresponded, sometimes prolifically, as they developed their own publications. When science and medicine formed the subject matter of a book and a social movement, direct author-to-author communication fostered translations, new texts, and strategies for negotiating the conflicts inherent in cultural change.

There is also the existence, in these authors' works, of their imagined colloquies with their readers. In his overview of the ways that books are circulated, Darnton has observed that "reading remains the most difficult stage to study in the circuit that books follow."[22] The problem is particularly true of books on sensitive subjects, and it is complicated further by young readers whose conduct was scrutinized for signs of dangerous activity. Strong prescriptive statements about youthful health and reading, always a factor in this Progressive Era information campaign, were articulated with increasing fervor as adults confronted the dilemma of actual young readers. The deceptively charming tableau of children playing school by "spelling out the long words" found in booklets on the "private diseases of men" and the discovery of a too-interested ten-year-old boy studying a pamphlet on women's health hidden in his schoolbook rationalized the scrutiny of what young people read.[23] Mikki Smith has observed that the communications circuit omits the nature of parental and librarians' involvement in selecting books for young readers, and anecdotes about young people's use of sexual health texts confirm that adult intervention was a shaping factor in youthful information access.[24]

It can hardly be unsurprising, then, that few if any readers left margin-alia or other obvious signs of their responses to these sexual health texts. A strikingly few exceptions reside in the Kinsey Institute's library, where one copy of *What a Young Woman Ought to Know* bears a faintly penciled vertical line accompanied by the letter "M" in the margin next to passages describing the evils of masturbation, though it is all but impossible to know whether these marks were made by a contemporary reader or a subsequent researcher.[25] Other titles from the Self and Sex Series in the Institute's library also indicate that a title was passed from reader to reader by the addition of names on end papers, and a few particular passages—seldom intensely personal or suggestive—were consulted.[26] Far more often, pages remain unmarked, with only the bindings and the covers showing wear. Cues about the anticipated contexts in which young people would read, however, were numerous.

Knowing the adolescent was very much the project of these writers, who tended to construct idealized notions of readership, and in time, the young reader became a recognizable type. As if to assure parents who worried that their own children might be harmed by inappropriate knowledge, authors established the image of the well-mannered and intelligent but not unduly curious child as a trope in these texts. The model child, captured in print, was a subtle marketing ploy, an implicit promise that the ideas espoused in the text would produce an obedient and thoughtful child, whose character was formed by parentally approved reading. It was a sharp and intentional contrast to the strategy used by one lesser-known pamphlet, which contained the story of an actual young woman whose premarital romance ended in infection and hospitalization.[27] Whether directly addressed or described as a character in a didactic narrative, readers were purposively invoked in the text.

Admittedly, numerous scholars argue that we cannot rely on portraits of implied readers.[28] Yet for hygiene treatises, these are often the only way long-ago readers remain available to us, and their images communicate much. It is significant that as inscribed in the pages of hygiene treatises, readers enjoyed both tangible and intangible resources. Financially secure and cared for by a loving family, the young readers envisaged in these texts lived, if not in a healthy, rural environment, then in a place where it was at least possible to walk in parks and gardens. They looked at plants and through microscopes. The readers addressed by hygiene authors had pets, friends, and eventually, suitable romantic attachments. They quietly evoked, too, the eugenic norms that many proponents of hygiene information endorsed. Beyond the pages of these treatises, these idealized readers seemed to look to futures rosy with promises of health and happiness.

It was not, however, an unconditional future. To secure the health of one's child, one relied on the right books. All who wrote about reproductive health did so believing that reading could be a healthful behavior and a prophylactic, easily the most effective prevention against lethal disease. Few authors spoke as frankly, and yet with as much restraint, as Fournier did, but he recognized that he must include parents as readers of the informative booklets intended as a public health measure. Stall, too, guided his audience to choose reading material with an eye toward shared, familial consumption. Would one's parents approve if they heard such words? "Never read, or listen to the reading of a book or paper which you might not ask your Mamma or Papa to read aloud with you," he directed young people, and his own series met this test.[29]

Others enlarged upon the notion that books with sensitive content should be read in the company of the family. In introducing a 1913 volume, *The Spark of Life,* Edward Bok advised that interactions between parent and child should shape the reading experience and that the text itself might even be omitted: "The value of the little book is, too, that it may be read by the parent, and from memory told to the child, or read to the child, or read by the child itself."[30] Similarly, Columbia professor Maurice Bigelow maintained a distinction between books that could endanger a young reader and those with healthful, helpful messages. It was not enough that young people be given books whose topics were safe, moral ones; he advocated that "the study of sex be brought into the light of day" with "good books" on the subject "read at the family fireside as properly as any other books."[31] Ruth Engs has described cycles of American health reform, which prioritized different prevention messages at different times; attitudes toward reading underwent similar shifts.[32]

The world was rendered darker and more complex as physicians' diagnostic skills outpaced their ability to cure the serious ailments whose lasting effects they began to understand more fully in the first years of the twentieth century. In the wake of one bold and decisive leader whose popular writing for adolescents gained readers around the world, others rushed to publish sexual health texts for young people. Authors responded to the uncertainties of science, first by introducing knowledge in the interest of prevention, then by proclaiming the young readers they strove to educate ever more innocent. Assuming that a pure readership required assurances about the rewards of rightful conduct was far less contentious than real induction into scientific reasoning. This vision gained a steadily increasing audience of individuals who were willing to spend their wages for information that once would have been unavailable unless illness forced them to visit a doctor.

Despite the availability of medical consultations, cures for sexually transmitted infections remained elusive, disputed, and finally, not universally accessible for many years. It would take almost as long for U.S. mass media outlets to agree to distribute sexual health information, prompted by government pronouncements. Until then, many concurred that the remedy for all that threatened young people was carefully sanctioned reading. Thus the modern practice of reading guidance emerged in connection with medical and reform interests in adolescent reproductive health, before it became the province of experts on children's literature, librarians and publishers among them. Regardless of whose authority governed the selection of texts, regulating young readers' appetites must have seemed a simpler task than constraining the flotilla of health texts that sold far and wide, permitting youthful innocence and a still maturing scientific knowledge to mingle.

These books proliferated, leaving traces in the cultural record and in individuals' possessions because medical science could not respond to disease effectively enough to ensure that patients would suffer neither short- nor long-term anguish. Fostered by international communication among medical practitioners and public health activists, prophylactic texts became more broadly available. As the emerging idea of adolescence became equated with sexual awakening, individuals who hoped to protect their children from harm purchased hygiene treatises. Scientific information and aggressive marketing alike encouraged commercial production of sexual health messages, despite laws that targeted a loosely defined concept of obscenity. Together, the promotion of books' decency and the privacy of mail-order and back-door purchases allowed individuals to read about sex with little sense of shame. Readers also bought the books we now find in attics and antiquarian collections because of libraries' responses to the emergence of these titles.

Librarians adopted the practice of reading guidance from medical professional and public health activists, while giving more attention to fiction than to critical health issues of the time. Commitment to information access was in flux during this period, and outside of urban areas like New York, states with progressive and well-funded private organizations like Connecticut, and cities and towns where universities were established, individuals could not depend on libraries to provide them with current health information. It has been claimed that Progressive Era librarians sequestered books on sex in closed stacks, denying access to anyone who could not demonstrate a legitimate reason for using a title.[33] This, certainly, is one story about the distribution of sexual health treatises. A leading publisher's perceptions of library borrowing as a force that countered purchases of his books and the documented placement of information about how to prevent venereal disease in libraries suggests another: libraries' acquisition and circulation of sexual health information was no more a unified phenomenon than was its authorship.

Numerous scholars have responded to Darnton's communications circuit by proposing shifts of emphasis or adding dimensions of the reading experience. Yet the reason so many individuals bought Stall's books or sent for Fournier's short treatises can only be derived from the extant copies of these works and the indications of their circulation. The transnational distribution of sexual health texts for adolescents hints at an intangible element, difficult to articulate in scholarly parlance. Of the questions we have asked about why books are created and shared, we have seldom reasoned about need, a notoriously fraught notion. American readers, and those abroad, responded to the unpredictability of texts' availability, the novelty of the information they contained, and an inability to predict that these new works would soon form a market in their own right. In other words, readers bought hygiene books to meet personal, even intensely private, senses of need. Readers may have hoped for the healthy families that Fournier and his colleagues wanted them to enjoy or the personal success that Stall and Hall implied could be theirs through living in accord with Christian precepts. The particular promises that appealed to readers cannot be clarified, while the dispersal of texts tells us that science and commerce pressed their cases for the need to read about health and the body, and that individuals who could respond to these innovative messages with pen or purchasing power did.

NOTES

INTRODUCTION

1. Allan Brandt, *No Magic Bullet: A Social History of Venereal Disease in the United States since 1880* (New York: Oxford University Press, 1987); Julian Carter, "Birds, Bees, and Venereal Disease: Toward an Intellectual History of Sex Education," *Journal of the History of Sexuality* 10 (April 2001): 213–49; John D'Emilio and Estelle Freedman, *Intimate Matters: A History of Sexuality in America* (Chicago: University of Chicago Press, 1997); Carl N. Degler, "What Ought to Be and What Was: Women's Sexuality in the Nineteenth Century," *American Historical Review* 79 (October 1974): 1467–90; Michel Foucault, *The History of Sexuality* (New York: Vintage Books, 1988–1990); Roy Porter and Lesley A. Hall, *The Facts of Life: The Creation of Sexual Knowledge in Britain, 1650–1950* (New Haven: Yale University Press, 1995); Thomas W. Laqueur, *Solitary Sex: A Cultural History of Masturbation* (New York: Zone Books, 2004); Jeffrey P. Moran, *Teaching Sex: The Shaping of Adolescence in the 20th Century* (Cambridge: Harvard University Press, 2000); Mary Odem, *Delinquent Daughters: Protecting and Policing Adolescent Female Sexuality in the United States, 1885–1920* (Chapel Hill: University of North Carolina Press, 1995); and John Parascandola, *Sex, Sin, and Science: A History of Syphilis in America* (Westport, Ct.: Praeger, 2008).

2. "The Saving Grace of Knowledge in Venereal Disease," *Medical News* 75 (4 November 1899): 589.

3. Daniel T. Rodgers, *Atlantic Crossings: Social Politics in a Progressive Age* (Cambridge: Belknap Press of Harvard University Press, 1998), 3.

4. This focus is not intended to dismiss the transnational circulation of social hygiene literature referred to in other research, such as R. Danielle Egan and Gail Hawkes, "Producing the Prurient through the Pedagogy of Purity: Childhood Sexuality and the Social Purity Movement," *Journal of Historical Sociology* 20 (December 2007): 444–61. The materials studied by Egan and Hawkes, however, were not generated by the network instigated by Fournier, nor do these works seem to share the purpose of disease prevention. As Egan and Hawkes themselves note, "As Historian Estelle Freedman illustrates, the ideologies of the 19th century literature on sexuality were highly variable, even within the same movement" (p. 458, note 6).

5. Jennifer Burek Pierce, "'Newly Invited . . . Into Government': Origins of Federal Government Information on Maternal and Child Health," *Journal of Government Information* 30, no. 5/6 (2004): 648–57; Jennifer Burek Pierce, "Science, Advocacy, and 'The Sacred and Intimate Things of Life': Representing Motherhood as a Progressive Era Cause in Women's Magazines," *American Periodicals* 18, no. 1 (2008): 69–95.

6. Margaret Deland, "I Didn't Know—," *Ladies' Home Journal*, March 1907, 9; Helen Keller, "Unnecessary Blindness," *Ladies' Home Journal*, January 1907, 14.

7. *Bulletin de la société française de la prophylaxie sanitaire et morale* (Paris: 1901–1909). Located at the Library of the New York Academy of Medicine (hereafter cited as NYAM).

8. James A. Secord, *Victorian Sensation: The Extraordinary Publication, Reception, and Secret Authorship of Vestiges of the Natural History of Creation* (Chicago: University of Chicago Press, 2001).

9. Roger Chartier, *On the Edge of the Cliff: History, Language, and Practices,* trans. Lydia G. Cochrane (Baltimore: Johns Hopkins University Press, 1997).

10. Andrew Scull, "The Fictions of Foucault's Scholarship," *Times Literary Supplement*, 21 March 2007; and Laura Hirshbein, review of *History of Psychiatry and Medical Psychology: With an Epilogue on Psychiatry and the Mind-Body Relation*, ed. Edwin R. Wallace IV and John Gach, *Bulletin of the History of Medicine* 83 (Summer 2009): 391–92. While Jeffrey P. Moran, in *Teaching Sex,* simply relocates the era of Foucault's proclaimed "discursive explosion" about sex to nineteenth-century America (p. 4), to question the accuracy and the relevance of Foucault's conclusions about sexuality to the analysis of historical medical discourse is far more common. For example, Roy Porter and Lesley Hall, in *The Facts of Life*, credit, within limits, Foucault's argument that "garrulity" rather than communicative restraint prevailed, but find, in the end, that his contentions oversimplify actual, subsequent discursive practices (p. 91, 105).

11. A related contention, in much the same language, is nonetheless made in the Foucauldian interpretation of hygiene literature in Egan and Hawkes, "Producing the Prurient," 444.

12. Michel Foucault, "What Is an Author?" in *The Book History Reader,* ed. David Finkelstein and Alistair McCleery, 2nd ed. (New York: Routledge, 2006), 291.

13. David M. Henkin, *The Postal Age: The Emergence of Modern Communications in Nineteenth-Century America* (Chicago: University of Chicago Press, 2007).

1. FRENCH ORIGINS OF INTERNATIONAL SEXUAL HEALTH COMMUNICATION WITH ADOLESCENTS

1. F. Trémolières, "The Scientific and Social Work of Alfred Fournier," *Prophylaxie antivenerienne* 23, no. 6 (1951): 230. Unless otherwise noted, translations are my own.

2. "Jean Alfred Fournier," *Journal of Neurology, Neurosurgery & Psychiatry* 65 (September 1998): 373.

3. Norman Howard-Jones, *The Scientific Background of the International Sanitary Conferences, 1851–1938* (Geneva: World Health Organization, 1975), 9.

4. Daniel Wallach and Gérard Tilles, "Henri Feulard (1858–1897): The Life and Works of the Secretary of the First International Congress of Dermatology," *International Journal of Dermatology* 37 (June 1998): 469–74; and "Society Proceedings," *Medical News* 81 (20 September 1902): 568.

5. "Délégués officiels des gouvernments" in *Conférence internationale pour la prophylaxie de la syphilis et des maladies veneriennes: Rapports preliminaires,* ed. Dubois-Havenith (Brussels: H. Lamertin, 1899), xvii–xxiv.

6. Homer Bostwick, *A Complete Practical Work on the Nature and Treatment of Venereal Diseases and Other Afflictions of the Genito-Urinary Organs of the Male and Female* (New York: Burgess, Stringer, 1848), 72–73. Located at the John Martin Rare Book Room, Hardin Library, The University of Iowa, Iowa City (hereafter cited as Hardin Library).

7. Bostwick (81, Hardin Library) urged that "The medical profession of the United States ought to come to the aid of public authorities, and the New-York Academy of Medicine would do well to offer as a prize question, the same that was not long since offered by the Society of Medical Sciences, of Brussels,—namely, 'What measures of medical police are best adapted to arrest the propagation of venereal diseases?'" His argument indicates awareness of medical and governmental responses to venereal disease in other nations, as well as the existence of concerned organizations, even if they were not specifically created to fight syphilis and gonorrhea.

8. "Society Proceedings," *Medical News,* 568.

9. Thomas W. Laqueur, *Solitary Sex: A Cultural History of Masturbation* (New York: Zone Books, 2003).

10. John H. Kellogg, *Plain Facts for Young And Old: Embracing the Natural History and Hygiene of Organic Life,* rev. ed. (Burlington, Iowa: I. F. Segner, 1886), 368, 408. Located at the Kinsey Institute for Research in Sex, Gender, and Reproduction, Inc., Indiana University, Bloomington (hereafter cited as Kinsey Institute).

11. John H. Stokes, *To-day's World Problem in Disease Prevention: A Nontechnical Discussion* (Washington, D.C.: U.S. Public Health Service, 1919), 128. Kinsey Institute.

12. Kellogg, Preface to *Plain Facts,* v.

13. Key theorists and historians undertaking this project have included Michel Foucault, *The History of Sexuality, Vol. 1: An Introduction* (New York: Pantheon Books, 1978); Steven Marcus, *The Other Victorians: A Study of Sexuality and Pornography in Mid-Nineteenth-Century England* (New York: Basic Books, 1966); and Peter Gay, *Education of the Senses: The Bourgeois Experience, Victoria to Freud,* Vol. 1 (New York: W. W. Norton, 1984).

14. Roy Porter and Lesley A. Hall, *The Facts of Life: The Creation of Sexual Knowledge in Britain, 1650–1950* (New Haven: Yale University Press, 1995).

15. Charles Burlureaux, *Pour nos jeunes filles quand elles auront 16 ans: Conseils discrets d'un médicin* in *Bulletin de la Société française de prophylaxie sanitaire et morale* 2 (Paris: J. Rueff, 1902): 523. NYAM.

16. Helen Lefkowitz Horowitz, *Rereading Sex: Battles over Sexual Knowledge and Suppression in Nineteenth-Century America* (New York: Alfred A. Knopf, 2002).

17. Porter and Hall, *Facts of Life*, 96.

18. Laqueur, *Solitary Sex,* identifies the early eighteenth century as a turning point in social attitudes toward masturbation, when the practice began to be stigmatized. See especially "Books, Reading, and the Solitary Vice," 302–58.

19. J. Darier, "Alfred Fournier, 1852–1914," *Annales de Dermatologie et de Syphiligraphie* (Chartres: Imprimerie Durand, July 1915), 16. Located at the Wellcome Library, London. Hereafter cited as Wellcome Library.

20. Georges Maurice Debove, *Alfred Fournier: Éloge prononcé a l'Académie de Médicine dans le séance annuelle du 11 Décembre 1917* (Paris: Masson, 1917), 5. Wellcome Library.

21. Alfred Fournier, "The Relation between Treatment in the Early Stage and Tertiary Syphilis" in *Selected Essays and Monographs: Translations and Reprints from Various Sources,* vol. 161, trans. Guthrie Rankin, M.D. (London: The New Sydenham Society, 1897), 433. Wellcome Library.

22. Alfred Fournier, *Prophylaxie publique de la syphilis* (Paris: Librarie J. B. Baillière et Fils, 1887), 6–7. Wellcome Library.

23. W. P. Lattimore, translator's preface of *Ricord's Letters on Syphilis* (Philadelphia: Blanchard and Lea, 1857), vii.

24. Ibid., v.

25. Prince Albert Morrow, *Social Diseases and Marriage* (New York: Lea, 1904), 25; and foreword to "Standard Statistics of Prostitution, Gonorrhea, Syphilis," Advance proof, not for publication (New York: American Social Hygiene Association, July 1919). Kinsey Institute.

26. Robert W. Taylor, *A Clinical Atlas of Venereal & Skin Diseases Including Diagnosis, Prognosis, and Treatment* (Philadelphia: Lea Brothers, 1889). Hardin Library.

27. Frederic Buret, *Syphilis in the Middle Ages and in Modern Times,* Physicians' and Students' Ready Reference Series, vol. 2 & 3, no. 15. Trans. A. H. Ohmann-Dumesnil (Philadelphia: F. A. Davis Company, 1895), 464. Kinsey Institute.

28. John H. Stokes, *Today's World Problem in Disease Prevention: A Non-Technical Discussion of Syphilis and Gonorrhea* in V.D. Bulletin 22 (Washington, 1919): 104.

29. Alfred Fournier, *De la contagion syphilitique* (Paris: Rignoux, Imprimeur de la Faculté de Médecine, 1860), 10.

30. See Judith Surkis, "Venereal Consciousness and Society," in *Sexing the Citizen: Morality and Masculinity in France, 1870–1920* (Ithaca, N.Y.: Cornell Uni-

versity Press, 2006), 189–96, for discussion of the Society's attitudes toward prostitution; see Charles Greene Cumston, "Prevention of Syphilis," *Journal of the American Medical Association* 47 (27 October 1906): 1375, for an American physician's statement about women forced into prostitution by low salaries.

31. Bostwick, *Complete Practical Work*, 81.

32. The medical phenomenon of innocent infection was discussed in the professional and general literatures. Accounts of the issue are found in Prince A. Morrow, *The Sex Problem: Social Diseases, Publicity, Sex Instruction, The Double Standard of Morality*, American Society of Sanitary and Moral Prophylaxis series, reprint 1 (New York: Society of Sanitary and Moral Prophylaxis, 1912), NYAM; and Edward Bok, *The Americanization of Edward Bok* (New York: Charles Scribner's Sons, 1965).

33. Alfred Fournier, "Relation between Treatment"; and L. Duncan Bulkley, "Unrecognized Syphilis in General Practice" in *Syphilis: A Symposium* (New York: E. B. Treat, 1902), 45, 49. Kinsey Institute.

34. Eugene Fuller, M.D., "A Few General Remarks on the Management of Syphilis," in *Syphilis: A Symposium*, 95.

35. Fournier, *Prophylaxie publique de la syphilis*, 6.

36. Debove, *Éloge*, 9.

37. Paul Marrin, *Le mariage théorique et pratique: son hygiène, ses avantages ses devoirs, ses misères*, Bibliothèque scientifique universelle series (Paris: Kolb, 1890).

38. Claude Quétel, *History of Syphilis* (Oxford: Polity Press, 1990), 149; and Theodore J. Bauer, "Half a Century of International Control of the Venereal Diseases," *Public Health Reports* 68 (August, 1953): 780.

39. Biographical essays on Fournier include "Jean Alfred Fournier (1832–1914)," *Journal of Neurology, Neurosurgery & Psychiatry* 65 (September 1998): 373; M. A. Waugh, "Alfred Fournier, 1832–1914: His Influence on Venereology," *British Journal of Venereal Disease* 59 (1974): 232–36; and Joseph C. Heffernan, "Alfred Fournier (1832–1914)," *Investigative Urology* 17, no. 3 (1979): 262–63.

40. Debove, *Éloge*, 3.

41. Alfred Fournier, *Syphilis et mariage*, 2nd ed. rev. (Paris: G. Masson, 1890), NYAM; and Michael Waugh, "Dermato-venereology: An Historical Perspective," *Journal of the European Academy of Dermatology and Venereology* 3 (1994): 551–54.

42. Fournier, *De la contagion syphilitique*.

43. Debove, *Éloge*, 4–5.

44. Eugène Brieux, "Pour les avariés," *Bulletin de la Société française de prophylaxie sanitaire et morale*, 3 (Paris: J. Rueff, 1902), 165, NYAM.

45. C. F. Marshall, translator's preface, *The Treatment of Syphilis* (London/New York: Rebman, 1906), xii; Debove, *Éloge*, 5; and Darier, "Alfred Fournier, 1852–1914," 15. Wellcome Library.

46. Fournier, *De la contagion syphilitique*, 9.

47. Debove, *Éloge*, 5.

48. Henri Rothschild, *Croisière autour de mes souvenirs* (Paris: Editions Émile-Paul Frères, 1932), 16, 305. Located at the Library of Congress.

49. Darier, "Alfred Fournier, 1852–1914," 16.

50. Ibid.

51. Quétel, *History of Syphilis*, 135.

52. Darier, "Alfred Fournier, 1852–1914," 15.

53. Peter Baldwin, *Contagion and the State in Europe, 1830–1930* (Cambridge: Cambridge University Press, 1999), 427; and Allan M. Brandt, *No Magic Bullet: A Social History of Venereal Disease in the United States since 1880* (New York: Oxford University Press, 1987), 5.

54. Debove, *Éloge*, 12.

55. Ibid., 10.

56. Brieux, "Pour les avariés," 165, NYAM.

57. Justin Sicard de Plauzoles, "Alfred Fournier et la Société de Prophylaxie Sanitaire et Morale," *Prophylaxie antivenerienne* 23, no. 6 (1951): 242–50.

58. Ibid., 245.

59. "Société de Prophylaxie Sanitaire et Morale," preface to Fournier, *Pour nos fils quand ils auront 18 ans* (Paris: C. Delagrave, 1905): n.p. Located at the Francis A. Countway Library of Medicine, Harvard University (hereafter cited as Countway Library).

60. Surkis, *Sexing the Citizen*, 190.

61. "Société de Prophylaxie Sanitaire et Morale," *Pour nos fils*, n.p. Fournier had articulated his intent to publish preventative sexual health information at the first international conference on syphilis in Alfred Fournier, "Danger Social de la Syphilie," *Rapports Preliminaires*, ed. Dubois-Havenith (Brussels: H. Lamertin, 1899), 36.

62. Alfred Fournier, "Nous allons procéder au vote de le titre sur la brochure de M. Burlureaux," *Bulletin de la Société française de prophylaxie sanitaire et morale* 2 (Paris: J. Rueff, 1902), 290. Other scholars have also commented on the Society's mission, drawing attention to its concerns with the regulation of prostitution. See, in this, Surkis, *Sexing the Citizen*, 193, and Alain Corbin, *Women for Hire: Prostitution and Sexuality in France after 1850*, trans. Alan Sheridan (Cambridge: Harvard University Press, 1990).

63. *Comité d'éducation féminine de la Société française de la prophylaxie sanitaire et morale* (Paris, n.d.). Box 203, folder 5, Social Welfare History Archives, Elmer L. Andersen Library, University of Minnesota, Minneapolis (hereafter cited as ASHA Records, Andersen Library).

64. The language here relies on Ronald E. Dahl, "Adolescent Development and the Regulation of Behavior and Emotion: Introduction to Part VIII," *Adolescent Brain Development: Vulnerabilities and Opportunities*, ed. Ronald E. Dahl and Linda Patia Spear (Annals of the New York Academy of Sciences: 2004), 1021:294–95.

65. Jeffrey P. Moran, *Teaching Sex: The Shaping of Adolescence in the 20th Century* (Cambridge: Harvard University Press, 2000).

66. Maurice Bigelow, *Adolescence: Educational and Hygienic Problems*, National Health Series (New York: Funk & Wagnalls, 1924), 1.

67. G. Stanley Hall, *Adolescence: Its Psychology and Its Relations to Physiology, Anthropology, Sociology, Sex, Crime, Religion and Education*, 2 vols. (New York: D. Appleton, 1904).

68. A. K. Rogers, "A Study of Adolescence," *The Dial, A Semi-Monthly Journal of Literary Criticism, Discussion, and Information* 37 (1904): 82.

69. Bigelow's refutation of Hall's thinking was explicit in *Adolescence: Educational and Hygienic Problems;* Thorndike's commentary is quoted by Ellen Condliffe Lagermann, *An Elusive Science: The Troubling History of Education Research* (Chicago: University of Chicago Press, 2000), 57, and Prince A. Morrow, "Should the Youth of This Country Be Instructed in a Knowledge of Sexual Physiology and Hygiene?" reprinted from *American Medicine* XI, no. 2 (13 January 1906): 55–57, Box 1, ASHA Records, Andersen Library.

70. Hall, preface to *Adolescence*, vol. 1, xiv.

71. Ibid., xv.

72. Ibid., x, xiv.

73. Bigelow, *Adolescence: Educational and Hygienic Problems*, 3.

74. G. Stanley Hall, "Co-Education," *Bulletin of the American Academy of Medicine* 7 (1906): 656; "Co-Education," Mind and Body: A Monthly Journal Devoted to Physical Education, Supplement to No. 156 (February 1907): 145.

75. Hall, preface to *Adolescence*, vol. 1, xiii.

76. Hall, *Adolescence*, vol. 1, 435.

77. Ibid., 324.

78. Fournier, *Pour nos fils*, 4. Countway Library.

79. Burlureaux, *Pour nos jeunes filles* in *Bulletin de la Société* 2 (Paris: J. Rueff, 1902): 504, NYAM.

80. "The Threat of Venereal Disease to the Working Class," *Bulletin de la Société française de prophylaxie sanitaire et morale* 2 (Paris: J. Rueff, 1902): 504, NYAM; and Charles Burlureaux, *Pour nos filles quand leurs mères jugeront ces conseils nécessaires* (Paris: C. Delagrave, 1905), 5–6, 12, Countway Library.

81. Remarks by M. l'abbé Fonssagrives, "Prophylaxie dans la classe ouvrière," *Bulletin de la Société française de prophylaxie sanitaire et morale* 3 (Paris: J. Rueff, 1902): 12, NYAM; and M. Granjux, "Prophylaxie dans les centres ouvriers," *Bulletin de la Société française de prophylaxie sanitaire et morale* 3 (Paris: J. Rueff, 1902): 285, NYAM.

82. Remarks by M. Pinard, "Prophylaxie dans les centres ouvriers," *Bulletin de la Société française de prophylaxie sanitaire et morale* 3 (Paris: J. Rueff, 1902): 286, NYAM.

83. William H. Schneider, "Puericulture and the Style of French Eugenics," *History and Philosophy of Life Sciences* 8 (1986): 265–77.

84. Joshua H. Cole, "'There Are Only Good Mothers': The Ideological Work of Women's Fertility in France before World War I," *French Historical Studies* 19 (Spring 1996): 639–72.

85. Sicard de Plauzoles, "Fournier et la Société," 247.

86. "Rôle prophylactique de l'éducation complète," *Bulletin de la Société française de prophylaxie sanitaire et morale* 3 (Paris: J. Rueff, 1902): 5, NYAM.

87. Meeting of October 10, 1903, *Bulletin de la Société française de prophylaxie sanitaire et morale* 4 (Paris: J. Rueff, 1904): 433, NYAM.

88. Executive Committee of the Pennsylvania Society for the Prevention of Social Disease, *Go Tell Other Girls: A Message from the Women of Philadelphia to the Mothers and Fathers of America* (Philadelphia: Pennsylvania Society for the Prevention of Social Disease, 1909), Countway Library.

89. Alfred Fournier, preface to Charles Burlureaux, *Pour nos filles quand leurs mères jugeront ces conseils nécessaires,* 3rd ed. (Paris: C. Delagrave, 1905), Countway Library.

90. Jill Harsin, "Syphilis, Wives, and Physicians: Medical Ethics and the Family in Late Nineteenth-Century France," *French Historical Studies* 16 (Spring 1989): 74.

91. Remarks by Charles Burlureaux, "Prophylaxie dans les centres ouvriers," *Bulletin de la Société française de prophylaxie sanitaire et morale* 3 (Paris: J. Rueff, 1902): 273, NYAM.

92. Alfred Fournier, "Les brochures," *Bulletin de la Société française de prophylaxie sanitaire et morale* 3 (Paris: J. Rueff, 1902): 500, NYAM.

93. Surkis, *Sexing the Citizen,* 197; Debove, *Éloge,* 14; see also H. Gougerot, "Alfred Fournier Intime," *Prophylaxie antivenerienne* 23, no. 6 (1951): 232–40. In addition to this ad hominem treatment of Fournier, Surkis castigated the man as misogynist, particularly in his views on the regulation of prostitution; it should be noted that Sicard de Plauzoles admits Fournier's regulationist tendencies, yet argues that his mentor's vision was for a "humanitarian" and "elevating" system. Fournier also, according to Sicard de Plauzoles, "condemned in the most severe terms the arbitrariness of the police des moeurs" (242–43).

94. Gougerot, "Alfred Fournier Intime," 235.

95. Ibid., 237.

96. John Thorne Crissey and Lawrence Charles Parish, *The Dermatology and Syphilology of the Nineteenth Century* (New York: Praeger, 1981), 141, 224.

97. Joseph-François Malgaigne, *Conseils pour le choix d'une bibliothèque: écrits pour une jeune fille* (Stamford, Conn.: Overbrook Press, 1936), Special Collections, Main Library, The University of Iowa, Iowa City.

98. M. Salmon, *Bulletin de la Société française de prophylaxie sanitaire et morale* 4 (Paris: J. Rueff, 1904): 34, NYAM.

99. Meeting of 1903, *Bulletin de la Société française de prophylaxie sanitaire et morale* 4 (Paris: J. Rueff 1904): 162–63, NYAM.

100. Meeting of 10 October 1903. *Bulletin de la Société française de prophylaxie sanitaire et morale* 4 (Paris: J. Rueff, 1904): 429–30, NYAM.

101. Charles Burlureaux, *Pour nos jeunes filles quand elles auront seize ans,* in *Bulletin de la Société française de prophylaxie sanitaire et morale* 3 (Paris: J. Rueff, 1902): 504, NYAM.

102. Charles Burlureaux, "Propagande individuelle," *Bulletin de la Société fran çaise de prophylaxie sanitaire et morale* 3 (Paris: J. Rueff, 1902): 496, NYAM.

103. "Peril venerienne dans la classe ouvrière," *Bulletin de la Société française de prophylaxie sanitaire et morale* 3 (Paris: J. Rueff, 1902): 502, NYAM.

104. Meeting of 4 July 1903, *Bulletin de la Société française de prophylaxie sani taire et morale* 4 (Paris: J. Rueff, 1904), NYAM.

105. Burlureaux, "Propagande individuelle," *Bulletin de la Société* 3 (Paris: J. Rueff, 1902): 496, NYAM.

106. Burlureaux, *Pour nos filles,* 13; and Fournier, *Pour nos fils,* 17.

107. Fournier, *Pour nos fils,* 8.

108. Ibid., 12.

109. Ibid., 18.

110. Trémolières, "Scientific and Social Work," 222, 223.

111. Ibid., 224.

112. Burlureaux, *Pour nos filles,* 6, 7.

113. "Rôle prophylactique de l'éducation complète," *Bulletin de la Société fran çaise de prophylaxie sanitaire et morale* 6 (Paris: J. Rueff, 1906): 6, NYAM.

114. Burlureaux, *Pour nos filles,* 30–31.

115. Henri Hayam in *Bulletin de la Société française de prophylaxie sanitaire et morale* 1 (Paris: J. Rueff., 1901): 288, NYAM.

116. Fournier, *Pour nos fils,* 15.

117. Burlureaux, *Pour nos filles,* 17.

118. Fournier, *Pour nos fils,* 14.

119. Brandt, *No Magic Bullet,* 16; and Angus McLaren, *Sexuality and the Social Order: The Debate over the Fertility of Women and Workers in France, 1770– 1920* (New York: Holmes & Meier, 1983), 155.

120. Burlureaux, *Pour nos filles,* 18; Fournier, *Pour nos fils,* 48.

121. Anne Summers, "Work in Progress: Which Women? What Europe? Jose phine Butler and the International Abolitionist Federation," *History Work shop Journal* 62 (2006): 215.

122. Brandt, *No Magic Bullet,* 11.

123. McLaren, *Sexuality and the Social Order,* 71.

124. Summers, "Work in Progress," 215, uses the phrase "international network ing" to describe Josephine Butler's late nineteenth-century campaigns oppos ing the regulation of prostitution.

125. Obituary of Alfred Fournier, *New York Times,* 25 December 1914.

126. Trémolières, "Scientific and Social Work," 230.

127. Sicard de Plauzoles, "Fournier et la Société," 247.

128. M. E. Devinat, "Conférences antiveneriennes," *Bulletin de la Société fran çaise de prophylaxie sanitaire et morale* 4 (Paris: J. Rueff, 1905), 163, NYAM.

129. Fournier, "Les brochures," *Bulletin de la Société* 3, 500, NYAM.

130. Burlureaux, "Propaganda individuelle," *Bulletin de la Société* 3 (Paris: J. Rueff, 1902): 495, NYAM. Emphasis original.

131. "Notre 5em Voeu," in *Bulletin de la Société française de prophylaxie sanitaire et morale* 3 (Paris: J. Rueff, 1902) 503, NYAM.

132. Alfred Fournier, *For Our Sons,* trans. Ernest A. Bell (Chicago: Night Church, c. 1917), 14. Although the SFPSM recorded the receipt of a letter from the U.S. War Department in 1902 that indicated the intent to distribute a translation of *Pour nos fils* to troops, there are no indications that it happened at that date. Alfred Fournier, *Bulletin de la Société française de prophylaxie sanitaire et morale* 3 (Paris: J. Rueff, 1902), 4, NYAM.

133. "Society Proceedings," *Medical News* 81 (20 September 1902): 568.

134. David J. Pivar, *Purity and Hygiene: Women, Prostitution, and the "American Plan," 1900–1930* (Santa Barbara, Calif.: Greenwood, 2001).

135. "Happy, Healthy Womanhood," V.D. series, 60 (Madison: Wisconsin State Board of Health/Copyright Social Hygiene Press, 1920). Located at the State Historical Society Library, University of Wisconsin, Madison.

136. John Hutchinson, preface to Alfred Fournier, *Syphilis and Marriage,* trans. Alfred Lingard (London: David Bogue, publisher to the Royal College of Surgeons, 1881), viii, Wellcome Library.

137. Alfred Fournier, *The Social Dangers of Syphilis: A Report Submitted to the International Congress at Brussells* [sic], *1899, for the Prevention of Venereal Diseases,* trans. Ernest A. Bell and Winfield Scott Hall (Chicago: The Midnight Mission, 1912). Located at the Library of Congress.

138. Translator's preface to Alfred Fournier, *The Treatment of Syphilis,* trans. C. F. Marshall (London: Rebman Limited; New York: Rebman Company, 1906), English translation of the 2nd edition, Wellcome Library.

139. Fournier, *Syphilis and Marriage,* trans. Alfred Lingard.

140. Brandt, *No Magic Bullet,* 11; "List of Delegates" in Emile Dubois-Havenith, ed., *Conférence internationale pour la prophylaxie de la syphilis et des maladies vénériennes,* 2 vols. (Brussels: Lamertin, 1899–1900).

141. Alfred Fournier, *Para Nuestros Hijos Cuando Tengan Dieciocho Años: Consejos De Un Medico* (Quito: Imprenta de la Universidad Central, 1904), II. Original Spanish translator unknown. Translated from Spanish to English by Rebecca Foster, 2006. Located at Government Information and Kent Cooper Services, Wells Library, Indiana University, Bloomington.

142. Fournier, *Pour nos fils,* 46–47.

143. Brandt, *No Magic Bullet,* 10.

144. Crissey and Parish, *Dermatology and Syphilology,* 141.

145. Mary Louise Roberts, *Civilization without Sexes: Reconstructing Gender in Postwar France, 1917–1927* (Chicago: University of Chicago Press, 1994), 184. One reviewer noted that "Cultural and political exchanges were becoming internationalized, and it would seem that the specificity of the French case needs to be contextualized" (367). See Christine Bard, review of Roberts,

Civilization without Sexes, Journal of Modern History 69, no. 2 (1997): 365–68.

146. Trémolières, "Scientific and Social Work," 230.

147. Denise Blanchier, "Faut-il parler aux enfants? Quand et comment?" *Comité d'éducation féminine de la Société française de la prophylaxie sanitaire et morale* (Paris, n.d.), Box 203, folder 5, ASHA Records, Andersen Library.

148. Roberts, *Civilization without Sexes*, 199–200.

2. INITIAL TRANSNATIONAL INTERSECTIONS

1. R. Danielle Egan and Gail Hawkes, "Producing the Prurient through the Pedagogy of Purity: Childhood Sexuality and the Social Purity Movement," *Journal of Historical Sociology* 20, no. 4 (2007): 443–61; Ruth C. Engs, *Clean Living Movements: American Cycles of Health Reform* (Westport, Ct.: Praeger, 2001); David J. Pivar, *Purity Crusade: Sexual Morality and Social Control, 1868–1900* (Westport, Conn.: Greenwood Press, 1973); and John D'Emilio and Estelle B. Freedman, *Intimate Matters: A History of Sexuality in America* (Chicago: University of Chicago Press, 1998).

2. Prince A. Morrow, "The Society of Sanitary and Moral Prophylaxis: Its Objects and Aims," in *Transactions of the Society of Sanitary and Moral Prophylaxis* 27 (New York: 1906). Kinsey Institute.

3. Ibid., 27.

4. Prince A. Morrow, "Report of Progress of the Society of Sanitary and Moral Prophylaxis," reprinted from *Social Diseases* (1912): 1. Box 1, folder 7, American Social Health Association Records, ASHA Records, Andersen Library.

5. E. L. Keyes, Obituary of Prince A. Morrow, *The Survey*, 12 April 1913: 76, ASHA Records, Andersen Library.

6. Theodore Tuffier, "The War against the Venereal Diseases in France," *Journal of the American Medical Association* 48 (October 1906): 1249.

7. Eugène Brieux, "Pour les avariés," *Bulletin de la Société française de prophylaxie sanitaire et morale* 3 (Paris: J. Rueff, 1902): 164, 167. NYAM.

8. Georges Maurice Debove, *Alfred Fournier: Éloge prononcé a l'Académie de Médicine dans le séance annuelle du 11 Décembre 1917* (Paris: Masson, 1917), 8. Located at the Wellcome Library, London.

9. Ibid.

10. Katie N. Johnson, "Damaged Goods: Sex Hysteria, and the Prostitute Fatale," *Theatre Survey* 44 (May 2003): 62n10. Johnson here documents the development from a handful of scattered performances at the turn of the century to more than 200 English performances by 1914.

11. Debove, *Éloge,* 8,

12. Richard Frederick Mundell, "Shaw and Brieux: A Literary Relationship," vol. 1, Ph.D. diss., University of Michigan, 1971, 6–7.

13. Barrett Harper Clark, "Eugène Brieux," in *Contemporary French Dramatists* (Cincinnati: Stewart & Kidd Company, 1916), 20.

14. Ibid., 19–20.

15. This characterization is by Clark, ibid., 29–31.

16. Ibid., 19.

17. Ibid., 20.

18. "Eugène Brieux (1858–1932)," in *The Continental Drama of Today,* ed. Barrett H. Clark (New York: Henry Holt, 1914), 157–58.

19. Clark, *Continental Drama,* 24.

20. Brieux, "Pour les avariés," *Bulletin de la Société* 3, 164, 167.

21. "Communications," *Bulletin de la Société française de prophylaxie sanitaire et morale* 3 (Paris: J. Rueff, 1902): 38–40. NYAM.

22. Clark, *Continental Drama,* 18.

23. George Bernard Shaw, preface to Eugène Brieux, *Damaged Goods/Les avariés: A Play in Three Acts,* trans. John Pollock (New York: Brentano's, 1912), v, ix. Printed for the Connecticut Society of Social Hygiene.

24. Loïc le Gouriadec, *Le mortel baiser: drame en 4 actes (édition populaire)* (Paris: Librairie Theatrale, 1927), n.p. box 23, folder France, ASHA Records, Andersen Library.

25. Shaw, preface to *Damaged Goods,* ix–x.

26. Eugene Brieux and George Bernard Shaw, *Three Plays by Brieux: Maternity; The Three Daughters of M. Dupont; Damaged Goods,* trans. Charlotte Frances Shaw, John Pollack, and St. John Hankin (Cambridge, Mass.: The University Press, 1907).

27. Johnson, "Damaged Goods: Sex Hysteria," 43; and Tuffier, "War against," 1249.

28. Upton Sinclair, press comments to *Damaged Goods: The Great Play "Les avariés" of Brieux* (Philadelphia: John C. Winston Co., 1913), 6–7; and Johnson, "Damaged Goods: Sex Hysteria," 44.

29. Eugène Brieux, *Damaged Goods/Les avariés: A Play in Three Acts,* trans. John Pollock (New York: Brentano's, 1912), 12.

30. Johnson, "Damaged Goods: Sex Hysteria," 45.

31. Ibid., 44.

32. Walter Clarke, "Dr. Prince Albert Morrow and His Aides," *Journal of Social Hygiene* 40 (May 1954): 192. Available from the Cornell University Home Economics Archive: Research, Tradition, History, hearth.library.cornell.edu/h/hearth (accessed Sepetember 26, 2010).

33. United States Office of Education, *Annual Report* (Washington, D.C.: GPO, 1913), 343.

34. Clarke, "Dr. Prince Albert Morrow and His Aides," 193.

35. Ibid., 192.

36. Thomas N. Hepburn, "Report of the Secretary" in *Report of the 3rd Annual Meeting of the Connecticut Society of Social Hygiene* (Hartford, 1913), 14. Located at the National Library of Medicine, Bethesda, Md. (hereafter cited as National Library of Medicine).

37. Clarke, "Dr. Prince Albert Morrow and His Aides," 192, 193.

38. "The Connecticut Society of Social Hygiene," *Social Diseases: Report of Progress of the Movement for Their Prevention* 3 (July 1910): 31–32, Box 3, folder 7, ASHA Records, Andersen Library.

39. Phineas H. Ingalls, "Address of the President," *Report of the 3rd Annual Meeting of the Connecticut Society of Social Hygiene* (Hartford: 1913), 11. National Library of Medicine.

40. *Report of the Commissioner of Education for the Year Ended June 30, 1912*, 1 (Washington, D.C.: Office of Education, 1913), 343.

41. Hepburn, "Report of the Secretary," 14. National Library of Medicine.

42. Ibid.; and Clarke, "Dr. Prince Albert Morrow and His Aides," 192.

43. "Medicine: New Magic Bullet," *Time*, 25 October 1943, www.time.com.

44. Upton Sinclair to George Bernard Shaw, 23 April 1913, Box 1, folder January–July 1913, Sinclair MSS, All Sinclair correspondence cited is courtesy of the Lilly Library, Indiana University, Bloomington.

45. Marcel Ballot to Upton Sinclair, 10 June 1913; and Upton Sinclair to Mme. Shaw, 27 June 1913. Box 1, folder January–July 1913, Sinclair MSS.

46. Sinclair to Shaw, 23 April 1913.

47. Upton Sinclair to John Pollock, 7 August 1913. Box 1, folder August–October 1913, Sinclair MSS.

48. Upton Sinclair to Marcel Ballot, 29 June 1913. Box 1, folder January–July 1913, Sinclair MSS.

49. Marcel Ballot to Upton Sinclair, 10 June 1913. Box 1, folder January–July 1913, Sinclair MSS.

50. Upton Sinclair to Marcel Ballot, 26 May 1913. Box 1, folder January–July 1913, Sinclair MSS.

51. Upton Sinclair to John Clark Winston, 6 August 1914. Sinclair MSS.

52. Sinclair to Winston, 6 August 1914.

53. Richard Bennett to Messrs. John Winston Co., 4 October 1913. Box 1, folder August–October 1913, Sinclair MSS.

54. Upton Sinclair to Eugène Brieux, 27 July 1913. Box 1, folder January–July 1913, Sinclair MSS.

55. Upton Sinclair to John Clark Winston, 13 August 1913. Box 1, folder August–October 1913, Sinclair MSS.

56. Bennett to Messrs. John Winston Co., 4 October 1913.

57. Richard Bennett to Messrs. John Winston Co., 8 October 1913. Box 1, folder August–October 1913, Sinclair MSS.

58. Upton Sinclair, preface to *Damaged Goods: The Great Play "Les avariés" of Brieux* (Philadelphia: John C. Winston Co., 1913), 5. Sinclair MSS.

59. Upton Sinclair, *Damaged Goods*, 33–34, 10, 23.

60. Thomas N. Hepburn recalled the first meeting of the American Society of Sanitary and Moral Prophylaxis as taking place on February 8, 1905. Clarke, "Dr. Prince Albert Morrow and His Aides," 191.

61. Keyes, Obituary of Prince A. Morrow, 76. ASHA Records, Andersen Library.

62. Clarke, "Dr. Prince Albert Morrow and His Aides," 188.

63. Dr. E. L. Keyes, notes of interview concerning Dr. Prince A. Morrow, 12 November 1946, transcript. Box 1, folder 1, ASHA Records, Andersen Library.

64. Ibid., 2, 1.

65. A biographical sketch of Morrow is provided by Charles Walter Clarke in "Dr. Prince A. Morrow, Humanitarian," in *Taboo: The Story of Social Hygiene* (Washington, D.C.: Public Affairs Press, 1961), 56; and Prince A. Morrow, *Social Diseases and Marriage: Social Prophylaxis* (New York: Lea Brothers, 1904).

66. Clarke, *Taboo*, 182.

67. Ibid., 21.

68. Claude Quétel, *History of Syphilis,* trans. Judith Braddock and Brian Pike (Baltimore: Johns Hopkins University Press, 1990), 136.

69. George Whiteside, "What Should We Teach the Public Regarding Venereal Disease?" *Journal of the American Medical Association* 47 (20 October 1906): 1253.

70. J. Riddle Goffe, "Discussion," *Transactions of the Society of Sanitary and Moral Prophylaxis* 118 (New York, 1906). Kinsey Institute.

71. Morrow, *Social Diseases and Marriage,* 42–23, v.

72. Papers that considered female sexuality were few. "That there is an instinctive shrinking on the part of girls and women, whatever their class, from any discussion of sexual matters goes without saying," asserted Dr. Margaret A. Cleaves, in "Should Education in Sexual Hygiene Be Given to Young Working Women?" *Transactions of the Society of Sanitary and Moral Prophylaxis* (New York, 1906): 112–13. Kinsey Institute.

73. Prince A. Morrow, "Foreword: A Plea for the Organization of a 'Society of Sanitary and Moral Prophylaxis,'" *Transactions of the Society of Sanitary and Moral Prophylaxis* (New York, 1906): 22, Kinsey Institute. Originally presented to the Medical Society of the County of New York, 23 May 1904.

74. E. L. Keyes, "The Sexual Necessity," *Transactions of the Society of Sanitary and Moral Prophylaxis* (New York, 1906): 42. Kinsey Institute.

75. Morrow, "Foreword," 19. Kinsey Institute.

76. "The Ages for Sex Instruction," *Transactions of the Society of Sanitary and Moral Prophylaxis,* 11 (New York, 1910). Kinsey Institute.

77. Morrow, "Foreword," 25. Kinsey Institute.

78. Morrow, *Social Diseases and Marriage,* 33, 34, 52, 46–70.

79. Allan Brandt, *No Magic Bullet: A Social History of Venereal Disease in the United States since 1880* (New York: Oxford University Press, 1987). Brandt observed, "In the early years of the twentieth century, some doctors continued to suggest that sex education might disrupt marriages, because women might come to understand the cause of many of their gynecological ailments. Physicians of the Progressive years, however, questioned the wisdom of the

femina tabula rasa in sexual matters." Yet attitudes toward women's sexuality varied depending, for example, on matters like nationality and culture, as well as the conditions that physicians witnessed in the venues in which they practiced. A number of historians, however, comment on the apparent relaxation of strictures against sexuality, particularly in print media, following World War I. Carl Kaestle presented some discussion of this in "Print Culture and Education in a Time of Rapid Social Change: Examples from A History of the Book in America" (*Education and the Culture of Print* conference, University of Wisconsin, Madison, 29 September 2006).

80. Prince A. Morrow, "The Sex Problem: Social Diseases, Publicity, Sex Instruction, The Double Standard of Morality" (New York: Society of Sanitary and Moral Prophylaxis, 1912). 8–9. NYAM.

81. Brandt, *No Magic Bullet*, 30.

82. Albert E. Carrier, "What Shall We Teach the Public Regarding Venereal Diseases?" *Journal of the American Medical Association* 47 (20 October 1906): 1250; and "Discussion," *Journal of the American Medical Association* 47 (20 October 1906): 1255.

83. Morrow, "Foreword," 23.

84. Constitution of *Transactions of the Society of Sanitary and Moral Prophylaxis*, 15 (New York, 1906). Kinsey Institute.

85. Prince A. Morrow, *Eugenics and Racial Poisons* in *Educational Pamphlets* (New York: American Society for Sanitary and Moral Prophylaxis, 1911–1912), 1–2. Kinsey Institute.

86. Max Oker-Blom, *How My Uncle the Doctor Instructed Me in Matters of Sex*, in *Educational Pamphlets* (New York: American Society for Sanitary and Moral Prophylaxis, 1911–1912), 2. Kinsey Institute.

87. American Society for Sanitary and Moral Prophylaxis, *Health and the Hygiene of Sex for College Students*, in *Educational Pamphlets* (New York: American Society for Sanitary and Moral Prophylaxis, 1911–1912), 2. Translated by Pnina Shachaf, Indiana University, 2007. Kinsey Institute.

88. Rose Woodallen Chapman to Mary Cobb, 2 September 1909. Box 1, folder 4, ASHA Records, Andersen Library.

89. Ibid.

90. Prince A. Morrow, "Education within the Medical Profession," *Medical News* 86 (24 June 1905): 1153. ASHA Records, Andersen Library.

91. Prince A. Morrow, "Report of Progress," ASHA Records, Andersen Library.

92. Morrow, "Education," 1157.

93. Morrow, "Foreword," 25.

3. SOCIAL HYGIENE VS. THE SEXUAL PLAGUES IN INDIANA AND THE WORLD

1. Anna Garlin Spencer, "Milestones in Social Hygiene" typescript, 20 April 1930, 1, box 1, folder 1, ASHA Records, Andersen Library.

2. Robert N. Willson, "The Relationship of the Medical Profession to the Social Evil," *Journal of the American Medical Association* 47, no. 1 (7 July 1906): 29.

3. Among the sources giving the list of the first ten American social hygiene associations are Gertrude R. Luce, "History of Social Hygiene, 1850–1930," typescript, April 1930. ASHA Records, Andersen Library; and Committee on Literature of the Spokane Society of Social and Moral Hygiene, "Circular no. 7: Social Hygiene for Young Women," 2nd ed. (November 1910), pyropus.ca/personal/interesting/social-hygiene-for-young-women/text.html.

4. "The Public Health," *Monthly Bulletin, Indiana State Board of Health* 13 (May 1910): 56.

5. "Indiana Paid $3,341,454 to Maintain Her Unfortunates," *Monthly Bulletin, Indiana State Board of Health* 12 (May 1910): 55.

6. The economics of illness were discussed by authors including Willson, "Relationship of the Medical Profession," 29–32.

7. Daniel J. Kevles, *In the Name of Eugenics: Genetics and the Uses of Human Heredity* (New York: Alfred A. Knopf, 1985), x.

8. "Dr. Hurty and His Work," unidentified news clipping (25 February 1915), box 3b, folder 11, Papers of Dr. John N. Hurty, Indiana State Archives (hereafter cited as Hurty Papers).

9. Kevles, In the *Name of Eugenics*, 300–301.

10. For a discussion of the founding of the Indiana State Board of Health, see Clifton J. Phillips, "Public Health, Welfare, and Social Reforms," *Indiana in Transition: The Emergence of an Industrial Commonwealth, 1880–1920* (Indianapolis: Indiana Historical Bureau & Indiana Historical Society, 1968): 469–81.

11. "John N. Hurty," *National Cyclopaedia of American Biography* 22 (New York: James T. White, 1932), 370–71.

12. Hurty to Bennett M. Grove, 23 December 1907, box 3b, folder 11, Hurty Papers.

13. John N. Hurty, Course in Hygiene notebook, Indiana Dental College, 12 November 1924, box 3c, Hurty Papers.

14. Matt L. Haines to John N. Hurty, 13 March 1915, box 3b, folder 6, Hurty Papers.

15. State Health Leadership Initiative, *The Recruitment, Selection, and Retention of a State Health Official: A Guide for the Appointing Authority,* The Association of State and Territorial Health Officials brochure (Washington: ASTHO, 2000), www.statepublichealth.org (no longer available).

16. Alexandra M. Stern, "'We Cannot Make a Silk Purse Out of a Sow's Ear:' Eugenics in the Hoosier Heartland," *Indiana Magazine of History* 103 (March 2007): 6–7.

17. John Duffy, *The Sanitarians: A History of American Public Health* (Urbana: University of Illinois Press, 1990), 3.

18. James H. Madison, *The Indiana Way: A State History* (Bloomington: Indiana University Press, 1986), xiv.

19. "Diseased Children," *Monthly Bulletin, Indiana State Board of Health* 13, no. 1 (January 1910): 6–7.

20. "The Indiana Child Creed," *Monthly Bulletin, Indiana State Board of Health* 13 (November 1910): 136.

21. Shari Rudavesky, "Looking at the History of Eugenics in Indiana," *Indianapolis Star,* 13 April 2007.

22. Bennett and Feldman, "The Most Useful Citizen of Indiana: John N. Hurty and the Public Health Movement," *Traces of Indiana and Midwestern History* 12, no. 3 (2000) 38; and "Dr. Hurty," *Indianapolis News,* 10 February 1911.

23. Prince A. Morrow, "Results Achieved by the Movement for Sanitary and Moral Prophylaxis—Outlook for the Future," in *Transactions of the Society of Sanitary and Moral Prophylaxis* 97 (New York: 1910). Kinsey Institute.

24. John N. Hurty to Dr. A. L. Bramkamp, 27 September 1909, box 3b, folder 11, Hurty Papers.

25. Claude Quétel, History of Syphilis (Oxford: Polity Press, 1990), 149.

26. Charles Walter Clarke, *Taboo: The Story of the Pioneers of Social Hygiene* (Washington, D.C.: Public Affairs Press, 1961). Clarke notes that "by 1910 there were local or state societies in New York, Baltimore, Chicago, Milwaukee, Philadelphia, Spokane, Portland (Ore.), Denver, St. Louis, Jacksonville, California, Texas, Colorado, Connecticut, West Virginia and Mexico City," 58–59.

27. Maurice A. Bigelow, Ph.D., Sc.D., *Health Education in Relation to Venereal Disease Control Education* (New York: American Social Hygiene Association, 1941).

28. Madison, *Indiana Way,* 222.

29. John N. Hurty to Dr. Prince A. Morrow, 19 July 1909, box 3b, folder 11, Hurty Papers.

30. Clarke, *Taboo,* 58–59.

31. Hurty to Rev. J. W. Oborn, 31 January 1908, box 3b, folder 11, Hurty Papers.

32. John N. Hurty to Dr. C. S. Runnells, 23 January 1908, box 3b, folder 11, Hurty Papers.

33. John N. Hurty to J. M. Maxwell, 24 December 1907, box 3b, folder 11, Hurty Papers.

34. John N. Hurty to Dr. R. G. Shanklin, 13 January 1907, box 3b, folder 11, Hurty Papers.

35. John N. Hurty to Dr. Charles Curtis Wallin, 11 February 1908, box 3b, folder 11, Hurty Papers.

36. Irving Fisher Papers, Manuscripts and Archives, Yale University Library.

37. Hurty to Fisher, 23 January 1908. Hurty Papers.

38. John N. Hurty to Dr. A. E. Bulson, 15 February 1908, box 3b, folder 11, Hurty Papers; and "Lewis C. Walker," *Biographical Directory of the Indiana General Assembly* 1 (Indiana Historical Bureau, 1984).

39. Charles Taylor, "Lewis C. Walker," in *Biographical Sketches and Review of the Bench and Bar of Indiana* (Indianapolis: Bench and Bar Publishing, 1895): 269. Located in the Indiana Division, Indiana State Library, Indianapolis.

40. John N. Hurty to Prof. E. P. Kreutzinger, 5 February 1908, box 3b, folder 11, Hurty Papers.

41. Hurty to Runnells, 23 January 1908.

42. John N. Hurty to Prof. Stanley Coulter, 24 January 1908, box 3b, folder 11, Hurty Papers.

43. The founding purposes of the American Society for Sanitary and Moral Prophylaxis included containing the spread of sexually transmitted infection and prostitution, studying the means of doing so, collecting statistics, recommending prevention strategies, and organizing similar societies. See "American Society of Sanitary and Moral Prophylaxis" (transcribed Certificate of Incorporation. 1 February 1907, ASHA Records, Andersen Library).

44. John N. Hurty to Dr. Etta Charles, 17 January 1908, box 3b, folder 11, Hurty Papers.

45. John N. Hurty to Mrs. O. N. Guldlin, 7 February 1908, box 3b, folder 11, Hurty Papers.

46. *Social Hygiene vs. the Sexual Plagues* (Indianapolis: Indiana State Board of Health, 1910), 5.

47. John N. Hurty to Dr. H. H. Sutton, 26 December 1907, box 3b, folder 11, Hurty Papers.

48. John N. Hurty to Rev. D. E. Dangel, 30 December 1907, box 3b, folder 11, Hurty Papers.

49. Hurty to Wallin, 11 February 1908.

50. John N. Hurty to Livingston Farrand, 6 February 1908, box 3b, folder 11, Hurty Papers.

51. *Social Hygiene vs. the Sexual Plagues*, 16.

52. John N. Hurty to Moses F. Dunn, 6 May 1909, box 3b, folder 11, Hurty Papers.

53. Jason S. Lantzer and Alexandra Minna Stern, "Building a Fit Society: Indiana's Eugenics Crusaders," *Traces of Indiana and Midwestern History* 19 (Winter 2007): 4–11.

54. *Social Hygiene vs. the Sexual Plagues,* n.p.

55. John N. Hurty to Rev. R. W. Harlow, 24 February 1908, box 3b, folder 11, Hurty Papers.

56. Hurty to Bulson, 15 February 1908.

57. *Social Hygiene vs. the Sexual Plagues,* 4.

58. Ibid., 4, 18.

59. Ibid., 24, 31, 32.

60. John N. Hurty to Judge Ben E. Lindsey, 2 July 1909; John N. Hurty to J. M. Fuller, 27 July 1909, box 3b, folder 11, Hurty Papers.

61. John N. Hurty to Elizabeth B. Grannis, 31 January 1908, box 3b, folder 11, Hurty Papers; "National Purity Conference," *The Elementary School Teacher* 7 (October 1906): 100–103.

62. John N. Hurty to Prof. Irving D. Fisher, 8 October 1908, box 3b, folder 11, Hurty Papers.

63. Hurty to Charles, 17 January 1908.

64. John N. Hurty to Dr. George McCoy, 28 February 1908, box 3b, folder 11, Hurty Papers.

65. Robert P. Bigelow, "Harry Walter Tyler," *Isis* 39 (November 1939): 60–64.

66. John N. Hurty to Prof. W. T. Sedgwick, 23 January 1909, box 3b, folder 11, Hurty Papers.

67. John N. Hurty to Julia Huppert, 26 January 1909, box 3b, folder 11, Hurty Papers.

68. John N. Hurty to Edna Hays, 7 May 1909, box 3b, folder 11, Hurty Papers.

69. John N. Hurty to Rudolph Leeds, 4 February 1908, box 3b, folder 11, Hurty Papers.

70. John N. Hurty to Perry Edwards Powell, 27 September 1909, box 3b, folder 11, Hurty Papers.

71. John N. Hurty to E. L. Mendenhall, 1 February 1908; Hurty to Kreutzinger, 5 February 1908; John N. Hurty to Rev. Ernest A. Bell, 24 February 1909, box 3b, folder 11, Hurty Papers.

72. John N. Hurty to E. K. Mohr, 29 July 1908, box 3b, folder 11, Hurty Papers.

73. John N. Hurty to Dr. George N. Jack, 18 June 1909, box 3b, folder 11, Hurty Papers.

74. "Hygiene vs. Sexual Plagues," *Monthly Bulletin, Indiana State Board of Health* 12 (April 1909): 60.

75. Hurty to Hays, 7 May 1909.

76. Hurty to Fisher, 8 October 1908.

77. John N. Hurty to Dr. L. Lowenfeld, 15 June 1909, box 3b, folder 11, Hurty Papers.

78. Hurty to Lindsey, 2 July 1909.

79. John N. Hurty to Mrs. Nellie Grinslade, 17 February 1909, box 3b, folder 11, Hurty Papers.

80. John N. Hurty to Mrs. Ethel L. Morgan, 16 February 1909; John N. Hurty to J. M. Fuller, 24 July 1909; John N. Hurty to L. M. Grosjean, 30 August 1909, box 3b, folder 11, Hurty Papers.

81. John N. Hurty to Rev. T. G. Brashear, 17 February 1909, box 3b, folder 11, Hurty Papers.

82. Hurty to Morgan, 16 February 1909.

83. John N. Hurty to Mrs. M. R. Wells, 18 February 1909, box 3b, folder 11, Hurty Papers.

84. John N. Hurty to Judge Ben E. Lindsey, 15 June 1909; Hurty to Grosjean, 30 August 1909; John N. Hurty to Dr. B. J. Queen, 2 January 1909, box 3b, folder 11, Hurty Papers.

85. John N. Hurty to James E. Tower, editor of *Good Housekeeping,* 7 January 1908, box 3b, folder 11, Hurty Papers.

86. John N. Hurty to Henry Geisler, 16 January 1909, box 3b, folder 11, Hurty Papers.

87. John N. Hurty to Effa V. Davis, 15 January 1909, box 3b, folder 11, Hurty Papers.

88. John N. Hurty to Allen Rosencrans, 15 January 1909, box 3b, folder 11, Hurty Papers.

89. John N. Hurty to Rose Woodallen, 20 January 1909, box 3b, folder 11, Hurty Papers.

90. John N. Hurty to S. H. Stone, 14 January 1909, box 3b, folder 11, Hurty Papers.

91. Hurty to Huppert, 26 January 1909.

92. In 1912, publishing statistics for *Social Hygiene vs. the Sexual Plagues* were reported at 100,000 copies in *Annual Report of the U.S. Office of Education* (Washington, D.C.: GPO, 1912): 343. Given the lack of uncomplicated Indiana government figures and the ambiguous role of the ISSH, it is impossible to determine whether the figure is accurate, representing the continuance of the pamphlet with private funds, or whether Hurty's estimates in his correspondence undercounted the publications prior to the legislature's mandate that distribution relying on state funds end.

93. Dorothy Porter, *Health, Civilization, and the State: A History of Public Health from Ancient to Modern Times* (New York: Routledge, 1999), 195.

94. News clipping, *Terre Haute Star*, 18 February 1911; news clipping, *Lebanon Pioneer*, 16 February 1911, box 3b, folder 11, Hurty Papers.

95. Indiana Board of Health, "Public Health in Indiana," http://www.in.gov/ history (no longer available).

96. "'Cranks' a Great Savings to State," news clipping, 8 February 1915, box 3b, folder 11, Hurty Papers.

97. News clipping, 25 February 1915, box 3b, folder 11, Hurty Papers.

98. John N. Hurty to J. R. Marsh, 30 January 1908, box 3b, folder 11, Hurty Papers.

99. John N. Hurty to Dr. Cressy Wilbur, 17 February 1908, box 3b, folder 11, Hurty Papers.

100. Alexandra Minna Stern, "Making Better Babies: Public Health and Race Betterment in Indiana, 1920–1935," *American Journal of Public Health* 92 (March 2002): 742–52. Authors writing about *The Indiana Mothers' Baby Book* have offered a range of dates for its publication; a search of the OCLC WorldCat database (accessed 11 June 2008) lists libraries including the Indiana State Library which identify 1914 as the first publication date for this title. If cataloging dates were assigned accurately, the volume was reissued in 1919, 1920, and 1924.

101. "The Indiana Child Creed," *Monthly Bulletin, Indiana State Board of Health* 13 (November 1910): 136.

102. John N. Hurty to Katharine C. Greenough, 23 August 1922, box 3b, folder 11, Hurty Papers.

103. See Stern, "We Cannot Make a Silk Purse Out of a Sow's Ear," for discussion of these laws.

104. Timeline at "Fit to Breed: History and Legacy of Indiana Eugenics," Indiana University and Indiana State Archives, www.iupui.edu/~fit2brd.

105. David L. Cowen, "John Newell Hurty," *American National Biography* 11 (New York: Oxford University Press, 1999): 573.

106. The final repeal of Indiana eugenics legislation took place in 1974; see "Fit to Breed," www.iupui.edu/~fit2brd.

107. Bennett and Feldman, "The Most Useful Citizen of Indiana," 43.

108. "John N. Hurty," Indiana State Department of Health, www.in.gov/isdh (no longer available).

109. A. G. Christen, S. J. Jay, and J. A. Christen, "Dr. John N. Hurty, MD: Zealous Public Health Educator, Indiana Dental College (1881–1925)," *Journal of the History of Dentistry* 28 (March 2000): 3–9.

110. Cowen, "John Newell Hurty," 572.

111. Bennett and Feldman note Hurty's early role in sex education and the publication of *Social Hygiene vs. the Sexual Plagues* but do not indicate the complexity or scope of this effort. Bennett and Feldman, "Most Useful Citizen of Indiana," 42–43.

112. "John Newell Hurty," *National Cyclopaedia,* 370.

113. John N. Hurty to Rev. Oscar E. Allison, 23 February 1909, box 3b, folder 11, Hurty Papers.

114. "Dr. Hurty," *Indianapolis News,* 28 March 1925.

115. David Klinghoffer, "Indiana Had Ties to Darwin's Dark Side," *Indianapolis Star,* 11 February 2007.

116. Ruth C. Engs, *Clean Living Movements: American Cycles of Health Reform* (Westport, Ct.: Praeger, 2000).

117. Madison, *The Indiana Way,* 152.

4. WHAT YOUNG READERS OUGHT TO KNOW

1. Agnes Repellier, "The Repeal of Reticence," in *Counter-currents* (New York: Houghton Mifflin, 1916), 136, 137, 148, 159.

2. Obituary of Sylvanus Stall, *New York Times,* 7 November 1915.

3. Sylvanus Stall, *Successful Selling of the Self and Sex Series* (Philadelphia: Vir Publishing Co., 1907), 324, Available from the Baker Library Historical Collections, Harvard University (hereafter cited as Baker Library, Harvard); and Theodore Schroeder, "The National Purity Conference" (n.d.), Theodore Schroeder Collection, Special Collections Research Center, Morris Library, Southern Illinois University, Carbondale (hereafter cited as Schroeder Collection).

4. Stall, *Successful Selling,* 324, 261.

5. Sylvanus Stall, *How to Pay Church Debts: And How to Keep Churches Out of Debt* (New York: I. K. Funk, 1881); Sylvanus Stall, *Methods of Church Work: Religious, Social and Financial* (New York: Funk & Wagnalls, 1887).

6. "The Rev. Sylvanus Stall, of Lancaster, Pa., editor of 'The Lutheran Year Book,' is organizing a party to make a ten weeks' bicycle tour through Nor-

way and Sweeden [*sic*] this year, setting out about June 1." *Daily Inter Ocean*, 13 March 1887; "In response to a large demand, Rev. Sylvanus Stall, D.D., associate editor of the Lutheran Observer, Philadelphia, Pa., has in preparation a second volume of Five Minute Object Sermons to Children," *Southwestern Christian Advocate*, 10 October 1895; and Obituary of Sylvanus Stall, *Chicago Daily Tribune*, 7 November 1915.

7. Sylvanus Stall, *Bible Selections for Daily Devotion* (Philadelphia: Vir Publishing Co., 1896).

8. "Our New Home," *Successful Selling for the Retail Book Salesman* 16, no. 2 (1927): 4. Located at the New York Public Library (hereafter cited as NYPL).

9. "Bookmaker's Corner," *Southwestern Christian Advocate* 23 (December 1897):15.

10. Schroeder, "The National Purity Conference" (n.d.), Schroeder Collection.

11. The dollar price tag was strongly associated with popular fiction and nonfiction works in this era, and cheapness with immoral literature, as noted in Denning's analysis of dime novels: "William Wallace Cook . . . defends the morality of the nickel thrillers against the dollar 'best seller'—'a difference in the price of two commodities does not necessarily mark a moral difference in the commodities themselves.'" Michael Denning, *Mechanic Accents: Dime Novels and Working-Class Culture in America*, rev. ed. (New York: Verso, 1998), 22.

12. Judy Hilkey, *Character Is Capital: Success Manuals and Manhood in Gilded Age America* (Chapel Hill: University of North Carolina Press, 1997), 2.

13. "Something New!" *Successful Selling for the Retail Book Salesman* 16, no. 1 (1927): 17, NYPL.

14. Stall, *Successful Selling*, Baker Library, Harvard.

15. Theodore Schroeder to Dr. [Alice] Stockham, 5 December 1906, Schroeder Collection. Schroeder advised Stockham that in publishing "The Wedding Night" she ought to "insert in some logically appropriate place in the pamphlet [an] argumentative statement showing the necessity for such advice. In this I would recommend that you do not rely wholly upon yourself as authority but that you quote numerous authorities. . . . A prosecuting attorney, Judge or Jury after reading such statements from others than yourself would approach the reading of your contribution with an entirely different attitude of mind than if such matters were not first called to his attention."

16. Hilkey, *Character Is Capital*, 45.

17. Sylvanus Stall, *What a Young Man Ought to Know, New Revised Edition* (Philadelphia: Vir Publishing Co., 1904).

18. Mary Wood-Allen, *What a Young Woman Ought to Know* (Philadelphia: Vir Publishing Co., 1898), n.p.

19. Ibid.

20. Christabelle Sethna, "Men, Sex, and Education: The Ontario Women's Temperance Union and Children's Sex Education, 1900–20," *Ontario History* 88

(September 1996): 185–206, has described Stall's books as forming a "best-selling" series, although no information is provided to substantiate this description. Stall's works appeared in lists of books received for review at prominent contemporary publications, but those who offered best-seller lists in the United States did not identify his works on these lists. The door-to-door distribution of texts likely reduced the number of volumes sold through retail outlets that were used to generate these kinds of tallies. See also Stall, *Successful Selling*, 328, Baker Library, Harvard.

21. "The Yale Bowl," *Successful Selling for the Retail Book Salesman* 5, no. 1 (1915): 12–13, NYPL.

22. L. M. Cross, "A Mountain Two Hundred and Twenty Miles High," *Successful Selling for the Retail Book Salesman* 2, no. 2 (1912): 4–5, NYPL.

23. L. M. Cross, "A Roll of Paper 5,000 Miles Long," *Successful Selling for the Retail Book Salesman* 10, no. 1 (1920): 16–17, NYPL.

24. Hilkey, *Character Is Capital*, 235.

25. Aaron M. Powell, ed., *The National Purity Congress: Its Papers, Addresses, Portraits* (New York: The American Purity Alliance, 1896).

26. Sylvanus Stall, *What a Man of Forty-Five Ought to Know* (Philadelphia: Vir Publishing Co., 1901).

27. Sylvanus Stall, *What a Young Husband Ought to Know* (Philadelphia: Vir Publishing Co., 1928).

28. "Literary Notes," *Friends' Intelligencer* 55 (June 11, 1898): 421; and Rose Woodallen Chapman, *Dr. Mary Wood-Allen: A Life Sketch* (Chicago: Ruby I. Gilbert, 1908).

29. Chapman, *Dr. Mary Wood-Allen*, 33–35, 50.

30. "Notes about Books," *New York Observer and Chronicle* 79 (August 8, 1901): 190.

31. "Literary Notes," *New York Evangelist*, 21 June 1900; "Purity Books" ad in *The Independent . . . Devoted to the Consideration of Politics, Social and Economic Tendencies, History, Literature, and the Arts* 53 (Sept. 19, 1901): vi; and C. Howard Hopkins, *History of the Young Men's Christian Association in North America* (New York: Association Press, 1951), 385.

32. "National Purity Conference," *The Elementary School Teacher* 7 (October 1906): 100.

33. Sylvanus Stall, *What a Young Boy Ought to Know* (Philadelphia: Vir Publishing Co., 1897); Mary Wood-Allen, *What a Young Girl Ought to Know* (Philadelphia: Vir Publishing Co., 1897).

34. Stall, *Successful Selling*, 327, Baker Library, Harvard.

35. Edward Bok was quoted as saying, "Consider me most receptive to the books which I see are going to follow this one." Stall, *What a Young Boy*, n.p.

36. Review of *What a Young Man Ought to Know*, *New York Evangelist*, 10 March 1898.

37. Stall, *What a Young Boy*, 17.

38. Christine Pawley has remarked on the developing differentiation between youth and adult books that had yet to solidify in the 1890s. Christine Pawley,

Reading on the Middle Border: The Culture of Print in Late-Nineteenth-Century Osage, Iowa (Amherst: University of Massachusetts Press, 2001).

39. Stall, *What a Young Boy*, n.p.

40. Ibid., 19, 17.

41. J. B. Kerfoot, review of *What a Young Boy Ought to Know*, *Life*, 28 June 1906, 788.

42. Stall, *What a Young Boy*, n.p.

43. Carl Becker, quoted in Joel Dinerstein, "Technology and Its Discontents: On the Verge of the Posthuman," *American Quarterly* 58 (September 2006): 572.

44. Stall, *What a Young Boy*, 34, 35.

45. Ibid., 25–26, 28.

46. Wood-Allen, *What a Young Woman*, 87–88.

47. Chapman, *Dr. Mary Wood-Allen*, 19, 13.

48. Wood-Allen, *What a Young Girl*, 189.

49. Mary Wood-Allen, *What a Young Girl Ought to Know* (London: Vir Publishing Co., 1905).

50. Stall, *What a Young Boy*, 50–51.

51. Ibid., 60.

52. Ibid., 61–62.

53. Margaret Deland, "I Didn't Know—" *Ladies' Home Journal*, March 1907, 9.

54. "What Pupils Should Understand," *Transactions of the American Society of Sanitary and Moral Prophylaxis for the Year Ending May 31, 1908* 2 (New York: The Society of Sanitary and Moral Prophylaxis, 1908): 14.

55. Wood-Allen, *What a Young Girl*, 10.

56. Mary Wood-Allen, "Pamphlet," quoted in Stall, *What a Young Boy*, 65.

57. Wood-Allen, *What a Young Woman*, 198.

58. Ibid., 147.

59. Ibid.; Carl N. Degler has remarked that far from embracing Victorian notions of women's asexuality, Wood-Allen suggests that "women's sexual feelings were . . . dangerously easy to arouse": "What Ought to Be and What Was: Women's Sexuality in the Nineteenth Century," *American Historical Review* 79 (October 1974): 1474.

60. Wood-Allen, *What a Young Woman*, 148.

61. Theodore Schroeder to Rose Woodallen Chapman, 8 November 1906, Schroeder Collection.

62. "Educational," *Outlook* 61 (February 18, 1899): 414.

63. Havelock Ellis, *Studies in the Psychology of Sex: Sex in Relation to Society, Vol. VI* (London: F. A. Davis, 1910).

64. Stall, *What a Young Boy*, 83, 112, 123–24.

65. Review of *What a Young Boy Ought to Know*, *The Independent . . . Devoted to the Consideration of Politics, Social and Economic Tendencies, History, Literature, and the Arts* 49 (September 23, 1897): 19.

66. "Book Notes," *New York Evangelist,* 9 September 1897.

67. Wood-Allen, *What a Young Woman,* 228; and Stall, *What a Young Man,* 131.

68. Wood-Allen, *What a Young Woman,* 228.

69. Sylvanus Stall, *What a Young Man Ought to Know* (Philadelphia: Vir Publishing Co., 1903), 102.

70. J. P. Warbasse, "Discussion," *Transactions of the American Society for Sanitary and Moral Prophylaxis* 1 (New York: The Society for Sanitary and Moral Prophylaxis, 1906): 122.

71. Stall, *What a Young Man,* 100, 142.

72. Sylvanus Stall, *What a Young Boy Ought to Know* (Philadelphia: Vir Publishing Co., 1909), 180–81.

73. Ibid., 179, 182–83.

74. G. Stanley Hall to Theodore Schroeder, 11 July 1906, Schroeder Collection. Hall's letter, written during his presidency of Clark University and not quite two years following his major treatise on adolescence, describes the way he has "been so badly bitten and so sharply criticized for going too far in both speech and writing that I have grown timid," indicating something of the cultural attitudes that prevailed at this time.

75. Stall, *Successful Selling,* Baker Library, Harvard.

76. L. M. Cross, "Our Service to the Book Trade Is Appreciated," *Successful Selling for the Retail Book Salesman* 9, no. 1 (1919): 6, NYPL.

77. The pair's business travels are alluded to in "Birthday Greeting to Sylvanus Stall," *Successful Selling for the Retail Book Salesman* 2, no. 3 (1913): 7, NYPL; L. M. Cross, ed., *Successful Selling for the Retail Book Salesman,* vols. 2–17 (Philadelphia: Vir Publishing Co., 1912–1928), NYPL. Cross's death is noted in library holdings records attached to a final issue at the New York Public Library; and W. C. Everett, "A Study Class That Is Making Good," *Successful Selling for the Retail Book Salesman* 8, no. 2 (1919): 16. NYPL.

78. "How to Make Good as a Book Salesman," *Successful Selling for the Retail Book Salesman* 10, no. 1 (1920): 15, NYPL.

79. Stall, *Successful Selling,* 90, 76, 74–75, 72, Baker Library, Harvard.

80. Ibid., 82, 74, 77, 78, 89.

81. Ibid., 78, 297, 92, 105.

82. David Paul Nord, *Faith in Reading: Religious Publishing and the Birth of Mass Media in America, 1790–1860* (New York: Oxford University Press, 2004). Chapter 6, "How Readers Should Read," examines this issue.

83. Stall, *Successful Selling,* 84, Baker Library, Harvard.

84. Ibid., 129, 130, 151, 126.

85. Ibid., 96.

86. Chapman, *Dr. Mary Wood-Allen,* 32.

87. Stall, *Successful Selling,* 95, 53, Baker Library, Harvard.

88. Nord, *Faith in Reading,* 113, 120.

89. Stall, *Successful Selling,* 198, 199, 191, 190, Baker Library, Harvard.

90. Ibid., 77, 45, 48–49.

91. "To the Book Trade," *Successful Selling for the Retail Book Salesman* 16, no. 1 (1927): 18, NYPL.

92. L. M. Cross, "Business Outlook Is Good in U.S.A.," *Successful Selling for the Retail Book Salesman* 4, no. 3 (1914): 11; and "The Vir Business in 1920," *Successful Selling for the Retail Book Salesman* 10, no. 1 (1920): 10, NYPL.

93. L. M. Cross, "We Say So!" *Successful Selling for the Retail Book Salesman* 10, no. 1 (1920): 14, NYPL.

94. "A Telling Philadelphia Window," *Successful Selling for the Retail Book Salesman* 6, no. 1 (1916): 11, NYPL.

95. "American Baptist Publication Society," *Successful Selling for the Retail Book Salesman* 3, no. 2 (1913): 9, NYPL.

96. "Stall's Books the World Around," in Wood-Allen, *What a Young Woman,* n.p.

97. Beth Luey, "Translation and the Internationalization of Culture," *Publishing Research Quarterly* 16 (Winter 2001): 48.

98. Stall, *Successful Selling,* 21, Baker Library, Harvard.

99. Ibid., 16.

100. Neither Basil Mathews, *John R. Mott: World Citizen* (New York: Harper & Brothers, 1934), nor Kenneth Scott Latourette, *World Service: History of the Foreign Work and World Service of the Young Men's Christian Associations of the United States and Canada* (New York: Association Press, 1957) mentions this undertaking. Nor were Stall's titles included in a 1912 bibliography "of the best materials" on subjects including Sex Instruction; International Committee of the YMCA of the USA, *Principles and Methods of Religious Work for Men and Boys* (New York: Association Press, 1912), 166. See also Stall, *Successful Selling,* 240, Baker Library, Harvard.

101. Sylvanus Stall, "Foreign Translations of Stall's Books," *What a Young Man Ought to Know* (Philadelphia: Vir Publishing Co., 1904); and "Notes About New Books," *New York Observer and Chronicle,* 2 August 1900, 158.

102. "Notes About New Books," *New York Observer and Chronicle,* 2 August 1900, 158.

103. Stall, *Successful Selling,* 21, Baker Library, Harvard.

104. "Stall's Books," *Successful Selling for the Retail Book Salesman* 4, no. 3 (1914): 22, NYPL.

105. "The Large and Constantly Growing Sale," *Successful Selling for the Retail Book Salesman* 3, no. 2 (1913): 10; and L. M. Cross, "London as We Found It," *Successful Selling for the Retail Book Salesman* 9, no. 3 (1920): 17, NYPL.

106. "A Chart and Its Explanation: A Noticeable Decline in Works of Fiction," *Successful Selling for the Retail Book Salesman* 6, no. 1 (1916): 16–17, NYPL.

107. L. M. Cross, "The Books That Are Known," *Successful Selling for the Retail Book Salesman* 4, no. 1 (1914): 7, NYPL.

108. William J. Fielding, "What Every Young Woman Should Know," *Little Blue Book No. 655* (Kansas: Haldeman-Julius, 1924). University of Wisconsin Special Collections, Madison; Esquire, *What Every Young Man Should Know* (New York: Geis, 1962/1933).
109. Daniel J. Kevles, "The Secret History of Birth Control," *New York Times*, 22 July 2001, www.nytimes.com.
110. Fielding, "Young Woman," 4, 5, 18.
111. Ibid., 30.
112. Sylvanus Stall, *What a Young Husband Ought to Know, Revised and Enlarged* (Philadelphia: Vir Publishing Co., 1928); contrast passage is from Stall, *Young Man* (1904).
113. "A nation-wide campaign against the scourge of syphilis . . . ," *Reader's Digest*, March 1937, 14. It should be noted, however, that even this federal government campaign met with opposition from other agencies, as broadcasters refused to air speeches that named syphilis, citing decency regulations. See "Syphilis and Radio," *Time*, 3 December 1934.

5. BATTLING BOOKS

1. Paul S. Boyer, *Purity in Print: Book Censorship in America from the Gilded Age to the Computer Age*, 2nd ed. (Madison: University of Wisconsin Press, 2002), xii.
2. Section 7 of "The Duties of Physicians to Each Other and the Profession at Large," in *Principles of Medical Ethics* by the American Medical Association, 16 May 1903, www.ama-assn.org/ama/pub/about-ama/our-history/history-ama-ethics.shtml.
3. Boyer, *Purity in Print*, 25–26.
4. Sylvanus Stall, *The Social Peril* (Philadelphia: Vir Publishing Co., 1905), 157. Located at the Center for Research Libraries, www.crl.edu.
5. Preface, ibid., vi–vii.
6. Prince A. Morrow, *Social Diseases and Marriage: Social Prophylaxis* (New York: Lea Brothers, 1904).
7. Theodore Schroeder, "'Purity' Books Suppressed," in his *"Obscene" Literature and Constitutional Law* (New York: Da Capo Press, 1972), 62.
8. Morrow, *Social Diseases and Marriage*, iii, 81, 84–85, 25.
9. Stall, *The Social Peril*, 55.
10. Morrow, *Social Diseases and Marriage*, 21, 384.
11. Stall, *The Social Peril*, 321.
12. Attorney Theodore Schroeder offered a synopsis of this charge on the endpapers of a copy of *The Social Peril* that he owned. He wrote: "This book was the means of a threat from Anthony Comstock to prosecute Stall for 'obscenity.' Subsequently and before definitive action was taken an injunction was secured to prevent publication as an infringement of copyright on Prince Morrow's book, *Social Diseases and Marriage*."
    While Schroeder would offer varying and conflicting accounts of the events

surrounding Stall's publication of *The Social Peril,* his recollections of these events form the primary account of the conflict. Stall, *The Social Peril.* Center for Research Libraries.

13. Jerold S. Auerbach, introduction to *"Obscene" Literature and Constitutional Law,* xi.

14. David M. Rabban, "Theodore Schroeder," *American National Biography,* vol. 19, ed. John A. Garraty and Mark C. Carnes (New York: Oxford University Press, 1999), 430.

15. Theodore Schroeder to Alice Stockham, 5 December 1906. Schroeder Collection.

16. Theodore Schroeder to B. S. Steadwell, 17 August 1906, Schroeder Collection.

17. Sylvanus Stall to Theodore Schroeder, 27 August 1906, Schroeder Collection.

18. Theodore Schroeder, "National Purity Conference" (n.d.), 3, Schroeder Collection.

19. Schroeder marked these pages of his copy with notations and indicated, with his famous skepticism, these parts were "Declared 'Obscene' by Mr. Comstock." Stall, *The Social Peril,* 293–307.

20. Theodore Schroeder, "National Purity Conference" (n.d.), 2, Schroeder Collection.

21. "National Purity Conference," *The Elementary School Teacher* 7 (October 1906): 103.

22. Theodore Schroeder to B. S. Steadwell, 25 October 1906; and "Be it resolved" (n.d.), Schroeder Collection.

23. B. S. Steadwell to Theodore Schroeder, 10 November 1906, Schroeder Collection.

24. E. C. Henry to Theodore Schroeder, 20 December 1906, Schroeder Collection.

25. Rose Woodallen Chapman to Theodore Schroeder, 22 October 1906, Schroeder Collection.

26. A selection of this correspondence is represented by two letters: Anthony Comstock to Theodore Schroeder, 22 January 1906; and Theodore Schroeder to Anthony Comstock, 23 January 1906, both in Schroeder Collection.

27. Theodore Schroeder, "National Purity Conference" (n.d.), Schroeder Collection.

28. Mary Wood-Allen, "To The Daughter Dear," in *What a Young Woman Ought to Know* (Philadelphia: Vir Publishing Co., 1898), n.p.

29. Theodore, "National Purity Conference" (n.d.), 2.

30. Ibid., 3.

31. Rose Woodallen Chapman, *Dr. Mary Wood-Allen: A Life Sketch* (Chicago: Ruby I. Gilbert, 1908), 35; Winfield Scott Hall, *Instead of Wild Oats: A Little Book for the Youth of Eighteen and Over* (Chicago: Fleming H. Revell, 1912).

32. "Northwestern University," *Daily Inter Ocean,* 24 June 1887, 3, Issue 92.

33. "Gay Graduates," *Daily Inter Ocean,* 28 March 1888, 7, Issue 4.

34. "Echoes and News," *Medical News* 84 (June 18, 1904): 1182; "American Medi-

cal Temperance Association," *Bulletin of the American Medical Temperance Association* IV, 1 (November 1896): 24.

35. For a fuller biography of Hall and attention to his involvement with contemporary eugenics and with the U.S. military's Commission on Training Camp Activities during World War I, see Fokion Burgess, The Calculus of the Flesh (Brown University, 2008). My appreciation for Burgess's sharing this work while in progress, as well as other resources, critical perspective, and collegiality, is strong.

36. Winfield Scott Hall, "The Changes in the Proportions of the Human Body During the Period of Growth," *Journal of the Anthropological Institute of Great Britain and Ireland* 25 (1896): 21–46.

37. Hall's medical and physiology texts included the following titles: *A Laboratory Guide in Physiology, with Appendices on Organization and Equipment* (Chicago: Chicago Medical Book Co., 1898); *The Anatomy of the Central Nervous System of Man and Vertebrates in General* (New York: F. A. Davis Co., 1899); *A Text-Book of Physiology* (Philadelphia: Lea Bros., 1899); *Elementary Anatomy: Physiology and Hygiene for Higher Grammar Grades* (New York: American Book Co., 1900); *A Text-Book of Physiology, Normal and Pathological for Students and Practitioners of Medicine* (Philadelphia: Lea Bros., 1905).

38. Winfield Scott Hall and Henry Fox Hewes, *Oral Lesson Book in Hygiene for Use in Primary Grades* (New York: American Book Co., 1901); Winfield Scott Hall and Jeannette Winter Hall, *The New Century Primer of Hygiene for Fourth Year Pupils* (New York: American Book Co., 1901).

39. Winfield Scott Hall, *Sexual Knowledge: The Knowledge of Self and Sex in Simple Language* (Philadelphia: John C. Winston, 1913). Kinsey Institute.

40. Allan Brandt, *No Magic Bullet: A Social History of Venereal Disease in the United States since 1880* (New York: Oxford University Press, 1987), 49–50.

41. Quoted in Paul Popenoe, review of *Intimate Life of the Individual, the Family, the Society, and the Race* by Winfield Scott Hall (Chicago: Midland Press, 1926), *Journal of Social Hygiene* 13, no. 6 (1927): 349. Available from the Cornell University Home Economics Archive: Research, Tradition, History, hearth.library.cornell.edu.

42. Winfield Scott Hall, *A Manual of Sex Hygiene* (Chicago: Howard Severence Co., 1913). Kinsey Institute.

43. See William J. Robinson, ed., *Sexual Truths versus Sexual Lies, Misconceptions, and Exaggerations* (New York: The Critic and Guide Co., 1919).

44. William J. Robinson, "Our Sexual Misery," ibid., 30.

45. Havelock Ellis, *The Evolution of Modesty* (Philadelphia: F. A. Davis, 1900), 185.

46. Winfield Scott Hall with Jeannette Winter Hall, *Girlhood and Its Problems: The Sex Life of Woman* (Philadelphia: John C. Winston, 1919), 126–27.

47. Winfield Scott Hall, *Adolescence in Children's Foundation Work* (Philadelphia: John C. Winston, 1919), 317; and Maurice Bigelow, *Adolescence: Educational and Hygienic Problems* (New York: Funk & Wagnalls, 1924), 41, 43.

48. John D'Emilio and Estelle B. Freedman, *Intimate Matters: A History of*

Sexuality in America, 2nd ed. (Chicago: University of Chicago Press, 1997), 206.

49. Hall, *Girlhood and Its Problems,* ix.

50. Winfield Scott Hall, introduction to *Youth and Its Problems: The Sex Life of a Man* (Philadelphia: John C. Winston, 1919). Kinsey Institute.

51. See chapter 2 of Brandt, *No Magic Bullet,* for an account of the organizations that worked to develop social hygiene instruction for the U.S. military in the early twentieth century.

52. *Annual Report of the Surgeon General, U.S. Navy, Chief of the Bureau of Medicine and Surgery to the Secretary of the Navy* (Washington, D.C.: GPO, 1918), 172–73, 175.

53. David J. Pivar, *Purity and Hygiene: Women, Prostitution, and the "American Plan," 1900–1930* (Westport, Ct.: Greenwood Press, 2002), 210; and *Annual Report of the Surgeon General,* 116.

54. *Annual Report of the Surgeon General,* 215.

55. Bigelow, *Adolescence,* 3.

56. Hall, *A Manual of Sex Hygiene,* 9.

57. Popenoe, review of *Intimate Life of the Individual* by Hall, 348–49.

58. Arnold Dresden, "The International Organization of Intellectual Work," *American Review* 2, no. 1 (1924): 62.

59. Hall, introduction to *Youth and Its Problems,* 7.

60. Winfield Scott Hall, "The Adolescent," in *The Child, His Nature, and His Needs: A Survey of Present-Day Knowledge Concerning Child Nature and the Promotion of the Well-Being and Education of the Young,* ed. Michael Vincent O'Shea (New York: A Contribution of The Childrens Foundation, 1924).

61. "The First Contribution of the Childrens Foundation," *McClure's Magazine* 1 (May 1925): 50; and Eva B. Hansl, "Books for Parents," *The Bookman: A Review of Books and Life* 59 (August 1924): 737–38.

62. For discussion of the evolution of scientific thought on adolescence, see Crista De Luzio, *Female Adolescence in American Scientific Thought, 1830–1930* (Baltimore: Johns Hopkins University Press, 2007).

63. Popenoe, review of *Intimate Life,* 348–49.

64. Winfield Scott Hall, *Father and Daughter: A Story for Girls; Daughter, Mother, and Father: A Story for Girls; John's Vacation: What John Saw in the Country;* and *Chums: John and His Father Study Some Life Problems* (Chicago: American Medical Association: 1913).

65. Other duplications of content in Hall's work are discussed in Julian B. Carter, "Birds, Bees, and Venereal Disease: Toward an Intellectual History of Sex Education," *Journal of the History of Sexuality* 10 (April 2001): 242.

66. Max Oker-Blom, *How My Uncle the Doctor Instructed Me in Matters of Sex* in *Educational Pamphlets* (New York: American Society for Sanitary and Moral Prophylaxis, 1911–1912). Kinsey Institute.

67. F. N. Whittier to Mrs. John Storer Cobb, 20 July 1916. ASHA Records, Andersen Library.

68. Alfred Fournier, "Syphilis and General Paralysis," in *Selected Essays and Monographs: Translations and Reprints from Various Sources* (London: The New Sydenham Society, 1897). Wellcome Library, London.

69. "Did Syphilis Come from America?" *Medical and Surgical Reporter* 25 (16 December 1871): 554.

70. Alfred Fournier, *Syphilis et Mariage*, trans. Alfred Lingard (London, 1881), Wellcome Library, London,; Alfred Fournier, *The Treatment of Syphilis* 2nd ed., trans. C. F. Marshall (London: Rebman Limited; New York: Rebman Company, 1906), Wellcome Library, London.

71. Prince A. Morrow, translator's preface to Alfred Fournier, *Syphilis and Marriage* (New York: D. Appleton, 1880), iii.

72. Alfred Fournier, "Clinical Lecture on Syphilis in Relation to Marriage," trans. Charles W. Dulles, *Philadelphia Medical News* 9 (4 January 1897): 145–48.

73. Alfred Fournier, *En guérit-on?* (Paris: C. Delagrave, 1906); and Alfred Fournier, *Pour en guérir* (Paris: C. Delagrave, 1907). NYAM.

74. See, for example, "How and When to Give Mercury in Syphilis," *Medical and Surgical Reporter* 30 (21 February 1874): 170.

75. Fournier, *En guérit-on?*, 4.

76. Ibid., 8.

77. Ibid., 10–11.

78. Ibid., 19–20.

79. Ibid., 95–96.

80. Mark Helprin notes the nature of French copyright in *Digital Barbarism: A Writer's Manifesto* (New York: Harper Collins, 2009), 128.

81. "Can Syphilis Be Radically Cured?" *American Journal of Clinical Medicine* 13 (July 1906): 1332; George M. Katsainos, "Community Health," *Boston Medical and Surgical Journal* CLXXIV (17 December 1914): 926–27; J. Darier, "Alfred Fournier, 1832–1914," trans. John E. Lane, *Journal of Cutaneous Diseases Including Syphilis* 36 (January 1918): 493.

82. *Syphilis, Gonorrhea and Gonorrhoeal Opthalmia* (Rochester, N.Y.: Health Bureau, 1916), 6, 7. National Library of Medicine.

83. "Syphilis à toutes les periodes Paludism-Pian" and "Traitement de la syphilis par l'hydroxyde de Bismuth radifière" (n.p.) were just two of the advertisements in *An Exact Serology Guides the Treatment of Syphilis*, Pamphlet 5: Studies and Publications from Institut Prophylactique, trans. Dr. Daily M. O. Robinson with Adelaide B. Baylis (Paris: A. Malone et Fils, 1916). Box 203, Folder France, ASHA Records, Andersen Library.

84. *An Exact Serology*, Box 203, Folder France, ASHA Records, Andersen Library.

85. "Results of the Combined, Simultaneous Salvarsan-and-Mercury Treatment of Syphilis by Schmidt," *Medizinische Klinik* 18 (15 January 1922): 74–76. Typescript translated by J. Christian Bay, p. 11. National Library of Medicine.

86. "Objectionable Medical Advertisements to Be Excluded from the Mails," *Journal of the American Medical Association* 4 (4 June 1904): 1500.

87. A sustained discussion of this aspect of Comstock's work may be found in Nicola Beisel, *Imperiled Innocents: Anthony Comstock and Family Reproduction in Victorian America* (Princeton: Princeton University Press, 1997), 49–75.

88. Anthony Comstock, *Frauds Exposed; Or How the People are Deceived and Robbed, and Youth Are Corrupted* (Montclair, N.J.: Patterson Publishing Corp., 1880/1969), 5.

89. Ibid., 388–89. It perhaps is worth noting that Comstock himself disavowed any pretense of "literary excellence," 5.

90. Ibid., 433.

91. Ibid., "Tabular View of Results," 435.

92. Albert Neisser, "The Relation Between Treatment in the Early Stage and Tertiary Syphilis," trans. Frank H. Barendt, in *Selected Essays and Monographs: Translations and Reprints from Various Sources* (London: New Sydenham Society, 1897), 413.

CONCLUSION

1. The history of reading guidance for young people in the United States, particularly attitudes toward fictional works, is explained by Leonard S. Marcus, *Minders of Make-Believe: Idealists, Entrepreneurs, and the Shaping of American Children's Literature* (New York: Houghton Mifflin, 2008).

2. Several instances of product placement occur in the Self and Sex Series, including Sylvanus Stall, *What a Young Boy Ought to Know, New Revised Edition* (Philadelphia: Vir Publishing, 1909), 128; and Sylvanus Stall, *What a Young Man Ought to Know* (Philadelphia: Vir Publishing, 1897), 42–43, 275. Kinsey Institute.

3. One such recommended library for boys and young men was promoted by Mary Wood-Allen, *Almost a Man* (Cooperstown, N.Y.: Christ, Scott & Parshall, 1907), 99. Kinsey Institute.

4. American Social Hygiene Association, "What to Read on Social Hygiene," *Library Journal* 45 (1920): 1019–20. ASHA Records, Andersen Library.

5. Harry G. T. Cannons, "Sex Hygiene," *Bibliography of Library Economy, 1876–1920* (Chicago: American Library Association, 1927), 577. Ellen Geller, *Forbidden Books in American Public Libraries, 1876–1939: A Study in Cultural Change* (Westport, Ct.: Greenwood Press, 1984), discusses motives for library censorship, though without directly addressing health-oriented works.

6. John Shaw Billings to Secretary, American Social Hygiene Association. 11 December 1911. American Social Health Association Records, box 3, folder 2, ASHA Records, Andersen Library; "The Social Hygiene Bookshelf: A Selected List of Social Hygiene Books for Home and Public Libraries" (New York: American Social Hygiene Association, n.d.): 3, box 172, folder 13, ASHA Records, Andersen Library.

7. Thomas N. Hepburn, "Report of the Secretary," *Report of the Fifth Annual Meeting of the Connecticut Society of Social Hygiene* (29 November 1915): 9, box 3, folder 16, ASHA Records, Andersen Library.

8. J. G. Buhler to Dr. Prince A. Morrow, 16 October 1912, box 3, folder 2, ASHA Records, Andersen Library.

9. G. Stanley Hall, "How and When to Be Frank with Boys," *Ladies' Home Journal*, September 1907, 26.

10. Rose Woodallen Chapman, "How Shall I Tell My Child?" *Ladies' Home Journal*, May 1910.

11. Thomas S. Kuhn, *The Structure of Scientific Revolutions,* 3rd ed. (Chicago: University of Chicago Press, 1996); and Robert Darnton, "What Is the History of Books?" in *The Book History Reader,* ed. David Finkelstein and Alistair McCleery, 2nd ed. (New York: Routledge, 2006): 9–26.

12. Kuhn, *Structure of Scientific Revolutions,* 6.

13. Ibid.

14. Ibid., 19.

15. Daniel R. Weinberger, Brita Elevag, and Jay N. Giedd, *The Adolescent Brain: A Work in Progress* (Washington, D.C.: National Campaign to Prevent Teen Pregnancy, June 2005); Ronald E. Dahl and Ahmad R. Hariri, "Lessons from G. Stanley Hall: Conducting New Research in Biological Sciences to the Study of Adolescent Development," *Journal of Research on Adolescence* 15 (November 2005): 367–82.

16. Jeffrey P. Moran, *Teaching Sex: The Shaping of Adolescence in the 20th Century* (Cambridge: Harvard University Press, 2000), 12.

17. "Jane Addams Pleads for Wayward Girls," *New York Times,* 9 December 1911, 7; and Jane Addams, "Why Girls Go Wrong, In Which Miss Addams Presents 'The Only Path That Is Open to Us in America,'" *Ladies' Home Journal,* September 1907, 13–14. Gender issues in hygiene texts, particularly British publications, are discussed by Lesley Hall, "Venereal Diseases and Society in Britain, from the Contagious Diseases Acts to the National Health Service," in *Sex, Sin, and Suffering: Venereal Disease and European Society since 1870,* ed. Roger Davidson and Lesley A. Hall (New York: Routledge, 2001), 120–36; and Lesley Hall, "Hauling Down the Double Standard: Feminism, Social Purity, and Sexual Science in Late Nineteenth Century Britain," *Gender & History* 16, no. 1 (2004): 36–56.

18. "Jane Addams Pleads for Wayward Girls," 7.

19. Darnton, "History of Books," 9.

20. Paul Erickson, "Help or Hindrance? The History of the Book and Electronic Media," at the Media in Transition Conference, MIT (October 8, 1999), web. mit.edu/m-I-t/articles/erickson.html.

21. Darnton, "History of Books," 12.

22. Ibid., 16.

23. Edward Bok, "In an Editorial Way," *Ladies' Home Journal,* September 1907, 7.

24. Mikki Smith, "'It's good to know someone who cares': Real Teens and the Novels of Jeannette Eyerly" (unpublished paper, History of Readers and Reading, School of Library and Information Science, The University of Iowa, Spring 2006). In the author's possession.

25. Mary Wood-Allen, *What a Young Woman Ought to Know, New Revised Edition* (Philadelphia: Vir Publishing, 1905), 152, 157. Kinsey Institute.

26. Stall, *What a Young Boy Ought to Know, New Revised Edition* (Philadelphia: Vir Publishing, 1909). Kinsey Institute.

27. Pennsylvania Society for the Prevention of Social Disease, *Go Tell Other Girls: A Message from the Women of Philadelphia to the Mothers and Fathers of America* (Philadelphia: The Society, 1909). Countway Library.

28. Christine Pawley, "'Seeking Significance': Actual Readers, Specific Reading Communities," *Book History* 5 (2002): 143–60; Jonathan Rose, "Rereading the English Common Reader: A Preface to a History of Audiences" in *The Book History Reader,* ed David Finkelstein and Alistair McCleery, 424–39; and Roger Chartier, "Labourers and Voyagers: From the Text to the Reader," in *The Book History Reader,* 87–98.

29. Sylvanus Stall, *What a Young Boy Ought to Know, New Revised Edition* (Philadelphia: Vir Publishing,1905). Kinsey Institute.

30. Edward Bok, foreword to Margaret Warner Morley, *The Spark of Life: The Story of How Living Things Come into the World, As Told for Girls and Boys* (New York: Fleming H. Revell, 1913).

31. Maurice Bigelow, *Sex-Education: A Series of Lectures Concerning Knowledge of Sex in Its Relation to Human Life* (New York: Macmillan, 1929), 121–22.

32. Ruth C. Engs, *Clean Living Movements: American Cycles of Health Reform* (Westport, Ct.: Praeger, 2001).

33. Martha Cornog and Timothy Perper, "History of Libraries and Sexuality Materials," in *For Sex Education, See Librarian: A Guide to Issues and Resources* (Westport, Ct.: Greenwood Press, 1996), 35–47. Cornog and Perper's selective discussion of the development of sexuality materials for the general reader, however, omits medical developments and hygiene movements.

INDEX

Note: Page numbers in *italics* indicate photographs or illustrations.

JENNIFER BUREK PIERCE is faculty in the School of Library and Information Science at the University of Iowa, where she is also affiliated with the university's Center for the Book. She teaches courses in literature for young people, the history of reading, and research methods. Her first book, *Sex, Brains, and Video Games: A Librarian's Guide to Teens in the 21st Century,* was published by ALA Editions, and she developed and wrote the Youth Matters column for *American Libraries* magazine. Recently she was awarded a Jay and Deborah Last Fellowship in American Visual Culture at the American Antiquarian Society for research on the history of games and toys for children.